—Diseases and People—

MONONUCLEOSIS

Alvin, Virginia, and Robert
Silverstein

Enslow Publishers, Inc.

40 Industrial Road	PO Box 38
Box 398	Aldershot
Berkeley Heights, NJ 07922	Hants GU12 6BP
USA	UK

http://www.enslow.com

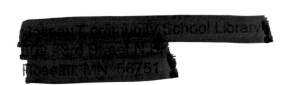

Library of Congress Cataloging-in-Publication Data

Silverstein, Alvin.
    Mononucleosis / Alvin, Virginia, and Robert Silverstein.
       p. cm. — (Diseases and people)
    Includes bibliographical references and index.
    ISBN 0-89490-466-3
    1. Mononucleosis—Juvenile literature. [1. Mononucleosis.
    2. Diseases.] I. Silverstein, Virginia B. II. Silverstein, Robert A.
    III. Title. IV. Series.
    RC147.G6S57 1994   93-48721
    616.9'25—dc20   CIP
                                            AC

Printed in the United States of America

10 9 8 7 6

Illustration Credits: ©1993 ATC Productions/Custom Medical Stock Photo, p.58; Bob Husth, pp. 6, 34; Centers for Disease Control, p. 22; Courtesy of the Children's Hospital of Philadelphia, p.17; ©1992 Custom Medical Stock Photo, p. 41; ©1993 Custom Medical Stock Photo, p. 51; ©1988 G.W. Willis, Biological Photo Service, p. 30; Larry Alpaugh, Tewksbury Photographers, p. 53; New Jersey Newsphotos, pp. 43, 79; Reprinted from "Epstein-Barr Virus Vaccines," by Andrew J. Morgan, in *Vaccine*, vol. 10, issue 9, 1992, by permission of the publisher, Butterworth Heinemann Ltd. © and Dr. Andrew J. Morgan, University of Bristol, pp. 69, 86; Simon Fraser, Hexham General Hospital/Science Photo Library, p. 45; St. Mary's Medical School, London, p. 36; University College Hospital, Ibadan/WHO, p. 61.

Cover Illustration: Cleo Photography/PhotoEdit.

Contents

Acknowledgments

The authors would like to thank Dr. Kevin Moore of DNAX and Dr. John A. Stewart of the division of viral disease of the Centers for Disease Control for their careful reading of the manuscript and their many helpful comments and suggestions.

Thanks also to Dr. Andrew J. Morgan of the University of Bristol (England), Dr. Stephen E. Straus of the National Institute of Allergy and Infectious Diseases, Maggie Bartlett of the National Cancer Institute, and all the others who kindly provided information and photographs for the book.

MONONUCLEOSIS

What is it? An infectious disease caused by the Epstein-Barr virus (EBV).

Who gets it? Mostly adolescents and young adults, of both sexes.

How do you get it? Through contact with infected saliva. Kissing is the most common route, but it can also be spread by sharing drinking glasses, toothbrushes, or other things that come in contact with the mouth.

What are the symptoms? At first general malaise, headache, fatigue, puffy, painful eyes, and loss of appetite; later sore throat, swollen lymph nodes (in the neck, armpits, and groin), general aches, and enlarged spleen or liver. (In children, EBV infection usually produces mild flu-like symptoms or no symptoms at all; in elderly patients symptoms include fever, tiredness, and abdominal pain.

How is it treated? Bed rest for one to three weeks; drinking fluids, eating a balanced diet; saltwater gargles for sore throats, acetaminophen for pain relief; strenuous exercise should be avoided as long as spleen enlargement persists. Most patients recover on their own within four to six weeks.

How can it be prevented? People infected with EBV in childhood are protected against infectious mononucleosis. There is no foolproof way for those not protected by a childhood EBV infection to avoid getting mono.

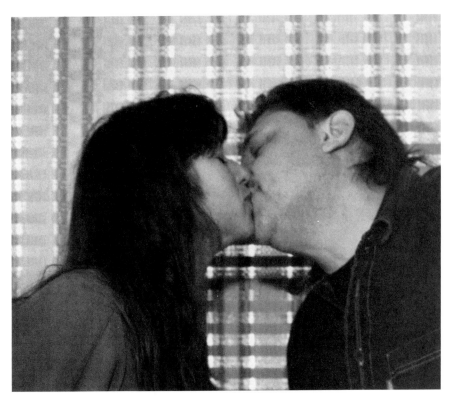

Mononucleosis is jokingly referred to as the "kissing disease."

1

The Kissing Disease

Matthew, a seventeen-year-old high-school junior in a Boston suburb, felt sharp pains in his eyeballs when he looked at his alarm clock one morning. When he looked in the mirror, he seemed normal except for a little puffiness around his eyes. He didn't think too much about it until two days later, when he had to come home early from school. He felt feverish and light-headed, his throat felt sore, there were swollen lumps in his neck, and he kept breaking out in a sweat. The doctor took a blood sample for tests and told Matthew to get some rest until the results were in. Matthew was getting ready for basketball season, and he didn't want to miss a day of his conditioning program. But when he tried to do his normal routine of one hundred sit-ups, he couldn't do more than ten.

After the doctor called the next day with the lab results, Matthew knew why he felt so wiped out. He had infectious mononucleosis—a flulike illness best known for striking teenagers and young adults. After resting in bed for ten days, Matthew felt much better. He wanted to get back to playing basketball in school. But the doctor felt Matthew's stomach and told him that his spleen was enlarged. (The spleen is responsible for storing blood and for producing disease-fighting white blood cells.) If he fell down or were bumped, his spleen might rupture—which would be very serious. Matthew had to wait another month before he could play with the basketball team. He was so excited about playing again that his first game back was the best of his career.[1]

Of all the diseases that people can get, mono (as infectious mononucleosis is often called) is the one illness that most people associate with teens and young adults. It is often jokingly referred to as the "kissing disease." Although kissing isn't the only way this disease can be spread, it is the most common way. Mono was first given this name by the chief physician at the U.S. Military Academy at West Point. He noticed that mono cases seemed to occur most often when cadets returned home from their Christmas holidays, during which they saw their girlfriends.[2]

"A kiss is just a kiss," an old song declares. But the "kissing disease" is nothing to sing about. Mononucleosis is hardly ever fatal, but each year it makes more than ten out of every thousand fifteen- to twenty-five-year-olds miserable for weeks or even months.[3] Sore throat, fever, and swollen glands are accompanied by a terrible tiredness that makes patients feel completely wiped out.

Mono tends to strike college students more than any other group of people. In fact, it is the second most frequent ailment prompting them to see a doctor. (Only upper respiratory infections cause more doctor's visits among this group.) The illness can be so devastating that many college students have had to drop out of school for a while, because they were unable to keep up with the work.[4]

Doctors have known about mono for about a hundred years. But they had no idea of what caused it until about twenty-five years ago, when it was discovered that mono is due to infection by a virus called Epstein-Barr virus (EBV). We now know a lot about the disease, but scientists still aren't sure why this virus can have very different effects on different people. Teens and young adults typically get infectious mononucleosis, but children infected by EBV usually have very mild symptoms, if any at all. And the same virus has been linked with cancer in some people. Recently, Epstein-Barr virus was believed to be the cause of a mysterious illness that made people extremely tired for months and months at a time.

As research continues, scientists hope to gain a better understanding of infectious mononucleosis and the virus that causes it. These studies may provide the keys to effective treatment for mono and a vaccine to prevent it.

2

The History of Mono

In the 1880s German doctors wrote about an illness that occurred mostly in children and spread to other family members. The patients had fever, sore throat, malaise, and swollen lymph glands. The illness was called "glandular fever," and it usually came on quickly and went away by itself after a short period of time. Traditionally, these German doctors were credited with being the first to describe infectious mononucleosis, although there were reports of illnesses with these symptoms dating back before the 1800s. However, experts today believe that most of the "glandular fever" patients described did not suffer from mono, but that the illness described was caused by other factors. One of the reasons for this doubt is that most of these German patients were children between five and eight years old, which is not the normal age group in which infectious mononucleosis develops.[1]

Nevertheless, the name "glandular fever" does refer to one of the most common symptoms of infectious mononucleosis—swollen glands. (The swollen lumps in the neck, groin, and armpits are not really glands; they are actually lymph nodes—tiny organs where disease-fighting white blood cells congregate, ready to go into action to help the body fight infections.)

In 1920 Dr. Thomas P. Sprunt and Dr. Frank A. Evans at Johns Hopkins University in Baltimore took blood samples from students with symptoms of swollen lymph nodes, fatigue, and fever. The doctors saw that these blood samples contained an unusually large number of a certain type of white blood cell called mononuclear lymphocytes. There weren't just more of these white blood cells—the cells also looked strange. They were larger than they were supposed to be, and the nucleus (the structure that directs the activity of the cell) was larger than normal. It is these "mononuclear cells" that give mononucleosis its name. Others had used the term infectious mononucleosis before Sprunt and Evans, but they were the first to use it to describe the disease we know today.

Mononuclear cells are also seen in other diseases, though, such as a type of cancer called leukemia. The symptoms of mononucleosis are similar to those of patients in the early stages of leukemia. At first doctors weren't sure whether patients with these symptoms had leukemia or mononucleosis. Often they had to wait for the patients either to develop symptoms of more advanced stages of leukemia, or to completely recover, if it was mono. Drs. Sprunt and Evans, however, pointed out that in mononucleosis the mononuclear cells were very similar to each other, but in leukemia the mononuclear cells were quite varied.

Sprunt and Evans had discovered how to tell the difference between mononucleosis and leukemia. Now mono patients no longer had to worry that they might be dying of leukemia. What they had was a much less serious illness, and it would get better by itself. However, just what was causing mononucleosis remained a mystery that would not be unraveled for fifty years.

Meanwhile, in 1932, a more conclusive way to diagnose mononucleosis was discovered. American physicians John Rodman Paul and Walls Willard Bunnell found that blood from humans with mono clumps (that is, the red cells gather together into irregular masses that can be seen under a microscope) when it is mixed with sheep blood. The sheep blood did not clump when mixed with blood from patients with other diseases. The clumping is due to a reaction by antibodies, special proteins designed to attack "foreign" chemicals, such as those on the surface of invading germs. (You might be wondering why scientists would mix human blood with sheep blood in the first place. In the 1920s, researchers had discovered that antibodies produced by one species of animal could be used to test for diseases in other species; so, this was not an uncommon procedure at the time.) The test, called the heterophile agglutination test (heterophile means "attracted to a different species"), has been refined over the years, but it remains one of the cornerstones for diagnosing infectious mononucleosis.[2]

Tracking Down a Mysterious Cancer

Researchers studying mononucleosis had a difficult time trying to find out what was causing the illness. In the 1930s and 1940s attempts were made to transmit the disease from infected people to animals, including monkeys, so that doctors could try to solve this puzzle. But these attempts were unsuccessful. By the early 1940s researchers began trying to transmit the illness to human volunteers; they used samples from throat washings, blood, lymph nodes, and feces of people with mono. Only rarely were they successful.

By the late 1950s most researchers studying mononucleosis thought it was caused by a virus. Some believed it might be caused by other microscopic organisms called protozoa. But no one was sure, and no one had been able to isolate the culprit. The mysterious cause was actually discovered through a series of lucky coincidences.

The first piece of the mononucleosis puzzle was uncovered in Africa in 1957. Dr. Denis Burkitt, a Scottish surgeon working in Uganda, was puzzled about strange tumors he kept encountering in African children. Huge swellings developed in some young children's jaws, and even when the tumors were surgically removed, the children died. When he checked local records, Dr. Burkitt found that the tumors had been occurring for more than fifty years, and they were rather common—they accounted for about half of all the childhood cancer in the area. Dr. Burkitt was surprised when a visiting doctor told him that this type of cancer was not found at all in South Africa.

Over the next three years, Dr. Burkitt sent out letters to other doctors and hospitals to track down where geographically the tumors occurred. "It was a part-time hobby, because I was employed full time as a government surgeon," notes Dr. Burkitt.[3] Then in 1961 he was given a grant and time off from work to venture on a ten-week, 10,000-mile "safari," investigating the disease in twelve different African countries. Dr. Burkitt found that the disease occurred only in specific areas. Trying to find a common denominator for all the places that it occurred, he finally concluded that the tumors developed in children living in places where disease-carrying insects were prevalent. Dr. Burkitt suspected the tumor might be caused by a virus carried by mosquitoes.

What Was Causing This Mysterious Cancer?

Meanwhile a British researcher, Dr. Michael Anthony Epstein of Middlesex Hospital in London, had heard Dr. Burkitt speak about the strange cancer, which had been named Burkitt's lymphoma. (Lymphomas are cancers of the lymphatic system, a network of vessels that drain excess fluid from the body tissues.) Dr. Epstein visited Africa and arranged for tumor samples to be sent to his laboratory so that he could search for the virus that was causing the disease.

First Dr. Epstein tried to get the tumor cells to grow in

the laboratory. Two years later, after he had been joined by a researcher named Yvonne Barr in 1963, he found the right conditions. In 1964, using an electron microscope, they discovered a virus present in the lymphoma cells. It looked like a member of the herpesvirus family (viruses that cause chicken pox, cold sores, and genital herpes), but it was not one that they were familiar with. So they sent a tumor sample containing the new Epstein-Barr virus to a former colleague, Dr. Klaus Hummeler, at the Children's Hospital of Philadelphia.

Dr. Hummeler had been in charge of the virus-diagnostic service at the hospital. By the time the virus samples arrived, however, the lab had lost its funding from the Pennsylvania Health Department and was no longer in operation. Hummeler turned to Werner and Gertrude Henle, a husband-and-wife team of researchers at Children's Hospital who specialized in the study of children's viruses.

Actually, the Henles were already interested in Burkitt's lymphoma. A year before, the chief surgeon at Children's Hospital, C. Everett Koop (who later served as U.S. Surgeon General) had returned from a trip to Africa with the news that the spread of Burkitt's lymphoma seemed to follow an infectious disease pattern. But when the Henles wrote to Dr. Burkitt, they were informed that many other researchers were already working on the problem. Now an opportunity to join the action had suddenly come up. "Klaus Hummeler came to our office, waving the bottles, to ask what should be done with them," says Werner Henle.[4]

15

Solving the Puzzle

The Henles quickly confirmed that the virus was a herpesvirus, one that had not previously been identified. In order to confirm that EBV was involved with Burkitt's lymphoma, they checked for antibodies for the virus in blood from children with Burkitt's lymphoma. (When the body is exposed to a virus or bacterium, it develops antibodies to fight the invader. So, if a blood sample contains antibodies against a particular virus, that means the body has been exposed to that virus.) All the victims had EBV antibodies in their blood.

But then the Henles discovered that nearly all healthy African children tested positive, too! In fact, nearly everyone in their lab also tested positive. But the Henles were able to link the virus to Burkitt's lymphoma, because children with the disease had concentrations of EBV antibodies that were eight to ten times higher than those of healthy children. Their bodies were trying hard to fight off the invading virus. Later EBV was also linked to a cancer common in adults in China and Southeast Asia, as well as Alaskan Eskimos.

The Henles believed that because the virus was so commonly found in people, it must be responsible for some common illness that affected many people. But what was the common illness?

The Henles discovered the answer completely by chance. A nineteen-year-old technician, Elaine Hutkin, was the only one in the lab who did not test positive for EBV antibodies. Late in 1967, she came down with chills, sore throat, and swollen glands, and felt very tired. A few days later she

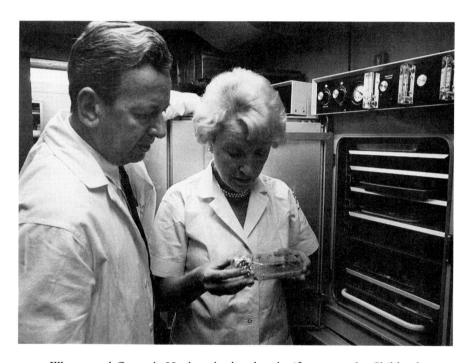

Werner and Gertrude Henle, a husband and wife team at the Children's Hospital of Philadelphia, were the first to discover that the Epstein-Barr virus causes mononucleosis.

developed a rash. The doctor said she had German measles. She came back to work after a week, but then grew sick again. The Henles did a blood test to find out what was wrong. This time the technician tested positive for EBV antibodies. In addition, her blood showed the mononucleosis cells that Sprunt and Evans had described nearly fifty years before. The lab technician did not have German measles—she had mononucleosis, and the Epstein-Barr virus seemed to have been the cause.

EBV had first been detected in cancerous tumors, and it now seemed to be involved in mononucleosis, a common cancerlike disease. It made complete sense. But the Henles needed more evidence before they were convinced. In New Haven, Connecticut, Dr. James Niederman of the Yale Medical School had been studying mono and collecting blood samples from hundreds of freshmen entering Yale since 1958. He had blood samples taken from students before they had mono, during the disease, and when they were well again. This was just what the Henles needed. Testing Dr. Niederman's samples, they found that the blood samples were always negative for Epstein-Barr virus before the illness, and always positive during and after the illness. "These findings led us to conclude unequivocally that the Epstein-Barr virus is responsible for at least one disease: infectious mononucleosis," the Henles wrote, and the mystery was officially solved.[5]

Over the years, scientists have learned a lot more about mono and the virus that causes it. Most of the knowledge about mono that scientists have gained has come from studying college students. In 1974, Dr. James Niederman reported the results of a four-year study of cadets who entered the U.S. Military Academy at West Point in 1969. He found that when the cadets arrived at school, 63.5 percent already had antibodies. Half of those who had not been infected had antibodies in their blood by the time they graduated four years later.[6]

Dr. Niederman's studies of students at Yale showed that by the late 1980s even more students had been exposed to EBV before they arrived at college—between 70 percent and 80 percent. Other studies have found that by age thirty-five, 90 percent of Americans are immune to the Epstein-Barr virus.

3

What Is Mono?

Joan felt miserable. "I remember coming down with something really strange," she recalls. "I don't usually like to give in to illness, but after a week of dragging myself around, it occurred to me that I might possibly be sick. Plus, I had these swollen glands in my neck.

"My doctor suspected that I had mono, but wanted to take a blood test to make sure it wasn't leukemia. I almost fainted when he said that. I had a couple of anxious days before the results of the blood test came back and, believe me, for once in my life I was delighted to be sick with something ordinary." Unfortunately, the doctor didn't have any medicine to prescribe. He just told Joan to rest until she felt well enough to go back to work.

"I was off work for a month, and when I went back to the office I took a lot of ribbing because I had the 'kissing disease.' Well, I suppose that's the way I got it, but I don't remember kissing anyone who was sick. It was sure a high price to pay. I felt weak and tired for a year afterwards."[1]

What Causes Mono?

Ninety percent of cases of mononucleosis are caused by the Epstein-Barr virus (EBV), which is a member of the herpes family. (This family also includes the viruses that cause cold sores, chicken pox, genital herpes, and birth defects.) Most of the remaining cases of mono are caused by another herpes-virus, cytomegalovirus.

Once a person is infected with a herpesvirus, it never really goes away. Herpesviruses get their name from the Greek word *herpeto,* which means "a creeping thing." (This is the same root as in "herpetology," the branch of science involving the study of reptiles and amphibians.) In a way, herpesviruses behave like snakes and salamanders. The viruses are able to lie hidden and inactive inside our bodies for long periods of time. When conditions are right, they "creep out" of hiding and become active.

Who Gets Mono?

Only humans and some primates can get infectious mononu-cleosis. Anyone from infants to the elderly can get mono, but it is mostly a disease of teens and young adults. About 70 percent to 80 percent of all cases occur in people between the ages of fifteen and thirty. High school and college students

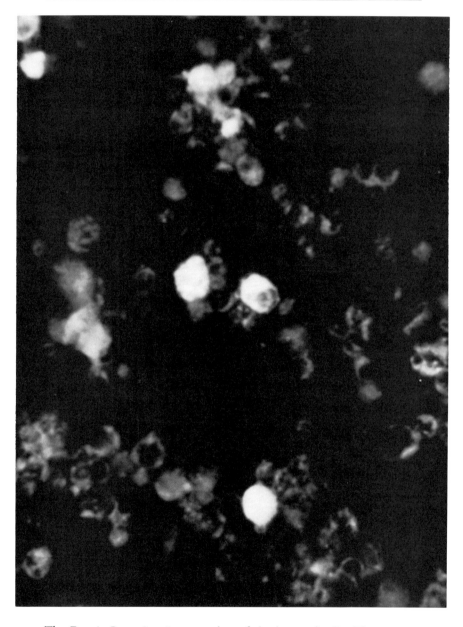

The Epstein-Barr virus is a member of the herpes family. The virus is responsible for 90 percent of all mono cases.

are the most likely to come down with infectious mononucleosis.

Actually, most people are infected with EBV during childhood. In the United States half of all children are infected by the age of five.[2] Nearly all the rest will become infected with EBV at some later time in their lives. (Scientists have estimated that 95 percent of all humans ultimately become infected.[3]) But not everyone who is infected with EBV gets infectious mononucleosis. Most children don't develop symptoms. Their bodies just manufacture antibodies against the virus. These antibodies stay in their blood all their lives, and protect them from ever developing infectious mononucleosis.

Adolescents who are infected are more likely to have mono symptoms. (With many viral diseases, symptoms are mild if the infection occurs in childhood, but they are more severe after people have reached maturity.) Researchers believe that the difference is in how the immune system reacts to the virus. Although adolescence is the prime time for developing the disease, only a small percentage of teens and young adults actually get infectious mononucleosis. This is because most young adults had already been exposed to EBV when they were children and are now protected against it.

Mono occurs slightly more often in males than in females. (By age thirty-five the gender differences have disappeared.) It peaks earlier in girls than in boys, though. Most females are fifteen to sixteen when they get mono; eighteen to twenty-three is the peak period for males.[4]

23

In the 1980s some reports claimed that the number of cases of mono in people over sixty had been increasing. Most public health officials disagree, however. They believe that doctors are just able to better diagnose the disease in the elderly now.

Most people get mono in the fall and early spring. Many infectious diseases of children and adolescents typically show a rise in the fall, when children return to school and are exposed to large groups of young people and the germs they are carrying. Students often develop mono during times of great stress, as well, such as during finals or before graduation. Mono does not occur in epidemics, but clusters of cases can occur.

ANNUAL CASES OF MONO BY AGE IN THE U.S.[5]

Age	Cases per 100,000
0–4	3–31
5–14	43–63
15–19	345–671
20–24	123–327
25–29	25–102
30–34	10–32
>34	2–4

Is EBV a New Virus?

The symptoms of mononucleosis were not described until a century ago. Moreover, the number of mono cases has been increasing over the years. According to a study in Connecticut, for example, there was a tenfold increase in mono cases between 1948 and 1967. Another study found the number of cases in the 1960s was 60 percent higher than in the 1950s.[6]

Do these observations suggest that the Epstein-Barr virus is relatively new in humans? Not necessarily. Scientists believe that there is a different explanation, involving changes in social and personal habits. As a society becomes more advanced, better hygiene and less crowded conditions make it harder for viruses to spread. Thus, exposure to the virus is delayed until people are older, when mono symptoms are more likely to develop. So the disease may be relatively new, but the virus that causes it has probably been around since ancient times.[7]

A Disease of Developed Nations

Infectious mononucleosis is essentially a disease of developed nations. In Third-World nations, most of the population still lives under conditions similar to those of past times, and most children there are still being exposed to the Epstein-Barr virus long before adolescence. In a study in Uganda, for example, 90 percent of children had been infected by the age of two or three; a study of Malaysian children found that 100 percent of children had been infected by age nine.[8] Actual cases of infectious mononucleosis are extremely rare in developing nations.

How Mono Is Spread

Mononucleosis is not easy to catch. It can be passed from one person to another through direct contact with infected saliva. Among infants, EBV might often be spread when one child plays with a toy another child has just had in his mouth.

In teens and young adults, the normal route is by kissing. Girls often date (and kiss) earlier than boys, which may be why the peak years for mono are earlier for girls than for boys. But mono is not just "the kissing disease." Sharing drinking glasses, silverware, or a toothbrush can also spread the disease. It can be spread by coughing, as well.

Blood transfusions can transmit EBV from one person to

HOW MANY PEOPLE GET MONO

- There are more than 100,000 cases of mono in the United States each year.

- 50 out of 100,000 Americans get mono each year.

- At colleges and universities the number may go as high as 300 to 1500 per 100,000—second only to upper respiratory infections.[9]

another, but health experts say that symptoms of the disease rarely develop under such conditions.[10]

A person can be infected only when someone who has the virus passes it to someone who has never been exposed. But less than 5 percent of those with mono can recall contact with someone else who had the disease. The Epstein-Barr virus is shed from the throat for up to six months after a person has mono. But people who have just gotten over infectious mononucleosis are not the only ones who spread the disease. From time to time, EBV becomes active in healthy people who had previously been exposed to the virus. It starts reproducing in the blood and in the lining of the throat. It is during these times that the virus is spread from one person to another. Studies have found that on any given day, between 15 percent and 25 percent of healthy people who have become "immune" to mono can actually spread the disease to someone who hasn't developed antibodies.[11] That means that when you're sitting in class, the chances are that up to one out of every four people around you are "shedding" EBV from the surface of their throats.

If so many people are contagious, it might seem odd that there are no mono epidemics. One reason is that the number of people who are susceptible is rather low at the time when people have the greatest chance of spreading the virus. Only about 20 percent of college freshmen have not been exposed to EBV. And among those in their thirties and forties, only 10 percent can catch it.[12] In addition, most people who come in contact with EBV do not develop the classic symptoms of mono. Overall, only half of adolescents and young adults exposed to EBV come down with mono symptoms. The rest either have no symptoms or such mild symptoms that they think it is just a cold.

Why Some People Are More Susceptible Than Others

Mono is most common among high school and college students, who may spend long hours studying, with tremendous pressure to succeed. Stress and fatigue have been shown to increase the chances of developing mononucleosis after exposure to EBV, because the body's immune defenses are lowered during such times. In studies of college students, 30 percent to 70 percent of those who were exposed to EBV came down with mono. But in similar studies with Peace Corps volunteers and military recruits, as few as 10 percent developed mono symptoms.[13]

What Happens in the Body

Mono mainly affects the lymphatic system. The virus first gets into the mouth and begins reproducing in the lining of the throat. The lymph system carries foreign invaders like EBV to special tissues where disease-fighting white blood cells called lymphocytes spring into action. But the Epstein-Barr virus infects one type of lymphocytes—the B cells that can produce antibodies—causing them to change, or mutate, and reproduce out of control. During mono, typically, one out of every ten B lymphocytes becomes "atypical." The nucleus of such a cell (the cell's control center) becomes enlarged, and there is more cytoplasm than normal inside the cell.

Other lymphocytes called killer T cells are alerted. They seek out and destroy the B lymphocytes infected with Epstein-Barr virus. This is what makes a person with mono sick—the body fighting its own cells. As the attack goes on, the battle sites (such as the lymph nodes) become enlarged and tender. Because the tonsils are masses of lymph tissue, they often become inflamed, causing a very sore throat.

Antibodies are usually produced before symptoms develop. When B cells are infected, they secrete many different antibodies, including heterophile antibodies. These are not directed against the virus and don't serve a protective function, but they do indicate that mono infection is present. (These antibodies react with antigens on the red blood cells of sheep, horse, and cattle.)

Finally, the T cells kill enough infected B lymphocytes so that the virus is under control. However, about one in a million B lymphocytes are still infected when the major battle is over. It's a kind of armed truce. Killer T cells continue to patrol the body, destroying infected B cells when they find them, but the struggle is never over. The virus periodically reproduces in throat cells and salivary glands and then can be spread from one person to another. "The Epstein-Barr virus has established a nearly perfect symbiosis with its human host ensuring the survival of both," researchers Werner and Gertrude Henle noted.[14]

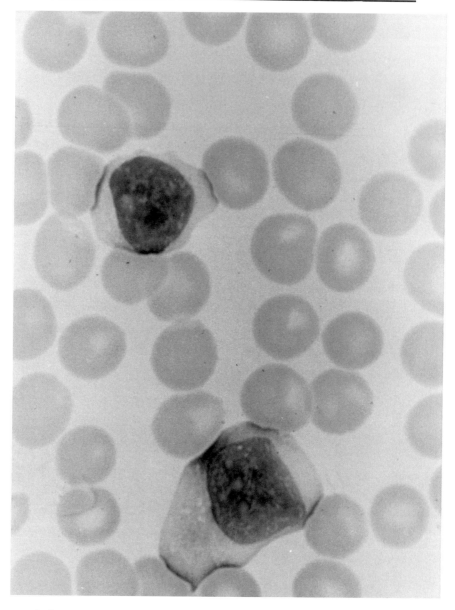

Infectious mononucleosis appears in the bloodstream, as shown here, by the presence of atypical lymphocytes.

Can You Get Mono More Than Once?

Most herpes infections can recur again and again throughout a person's lifetime. But infectious mononucleosis is different. Like other herpesviruses, EBV stays in the body for the rest of a person's life, but recurrences of mono are extremely rare and unusual. However, a relapse can occur as late as six to nine months after symptoms begin, if the illness was not totally brought under control the first time.[15] Nearly all of those who do have repeated monolike illnesses have immune systems that are not working properly, for example, AIDS patients or transplant recipients who are taking drugs to suppress the immune system. Or the person may be suffering from an attack of a virus that is not EBV but produces similar symptoms.

Cytomegalovirus—The Other Mono Virus

Cytomegalovirus (CMV) is a type of herpesvirus. "Cytomegalo" means enlarged cells; this virus may cause cells that it infects to become enlarged in a characteristic way. Only people can become infected with human CMV. Other strains of CMV appear in animals, but people cannot be infected by those.

Infection with CMV is very common. From 40 percent of all the adults in industrialized countries to 100 percent of adult populations in developing nations have been infected with and have developed antibodies against CMV.[16]

Most people who are infected by CMV never develop any symptoms. Those with weakened immune systems, such as people with AIDS, patients with cancer or with transplanted

31

organs, and the elderly, may develop more serious CMV infections such as lung diseases. A pregnant woman can infect her unborn baby. This may cause many different birth defects, including blindness, seizures, anemia, and brain damage.

In those with severe cases, the virus can cause different types of illness depending on the person's age. Newborn infants may have jaundice and be less than the normal weight at birth. In severe cases infants who are infected with CMV may become blind or deaf, suffer brain damage or even die. Infants infected during birth may develop symptoms three to twelve weeks after being born.

Young children infected with CMV may develop hepatitis (a destructive liver infection), with an enlargement of the liver. In older children and adults, the illness is often like mononucleosis or hepatitis.

CMV is excreted in saliva, urine, breast milk, semen, and cervical secretions, and so it can be passed from one person to another during sexual activity. It can also be passed when bodily fluids from an infected person pass through the mucous membrane of a body cavity, such as the mouth.

Blood transfusions are another method of transmission. When a patient develops mononucleosis after a blood transfusion, most often it is due to CMV. Those who become ill after a transfusion do so three to eight weeks later.

Once a person is infected, the virus may be shed for several years, but even after that the virus still remains in the body. If the person's immune system later becomes damaged, he or she may begin excreting CMV in bodily fluids again.

Symptoms of Mono

Once an adolescent or young adult who has not previously been exposed to EBV is infected, there is a 30 percent to 50 percent chance that mononucleosis symptoms will develop. Symptoms do not develop immediately after exposure, however. An incubation period lasts from two to seven weeks, during which the virus is attacking and multiplying and the body is mounting defenses against it—but the person is completely unaware of all this frantic activity.

Typically, mono develops slowly. The first symptoms are vague and easily mistaken for other illnesses, such as a cold or flu. The person just doesn't feel well and may complain of headache, tiredness, loss of appetite, chills, and puffy eyelids.

Gradually the symptoms become more severe as the body's lymphatic and disease-fighting systems are affected. The second wave of symptoms commonly includes a severe sore throat, fever (sometimes with chills), and general aches. Lymph nodes in the side and back of the neck, as well as in the armpits and groin, are swollen. The person may sweat excessively and be sensitive to bright lights. The exact combination of symptoms can vary, and the illness may be misdiagnosed at first as strep throat, German measles, hepatitis, syphilis, diphtheria, or leukemia. The typical mono symptoms usually last for one to three weeks, although they may be gone in as little as a few days or drag on for months.

Fever, which develops in about three-quarters of mono patients, typically goes up to 101 to 105 degrees. After about five days the body temperature usually returns to normal, but the fever may continue on and off for several weeks. (If high

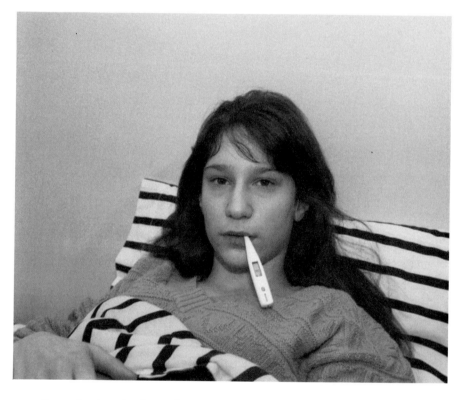

Fever develops in about three-quarters of mono patients, adding to the misery of the disease.

fever develops late in the illness, this is usually a sign of bacterial complications.)

Swollen lymph nodes range in size from a bean to a small egg, and are firm and painful if touched. The swelling slowly goes away over a few days or weeks.

About 50 percent of mono patients have enlargement of the spleen, which reaches a peak by the second or third week of the illness. About 20 percent have an enlarged liver, with liver problems occurring during the first three to five weeks. (The liver problems may cause jaundice, a yellowish tinge of the skin that goes away when the illness is over.)

About half of all mono patients have bumps on the tongue; one third have puffy, painful eyes; and one tenth develop a rash like German measles. Tonsillitis, difficulty in swallowing, and bleeding gums may develop. Coughing, nausea, and vomiting are other symptoms experienced by some mono patients.

Although most mono symptoms don't last too long, tiredness can persist for months. Most people feel well enough to go back to school or work after two to four weeks.

Occasionally, otherwise healthy people may develop very serious complications after EBV infection. These complications, which may be life-threatening, will be discussed in a later chapter.

Symptoms in the Elderly

Between 3 percent and 10 percent of those over age sixty have not developed Epstein-Barr antibodies. These people can get

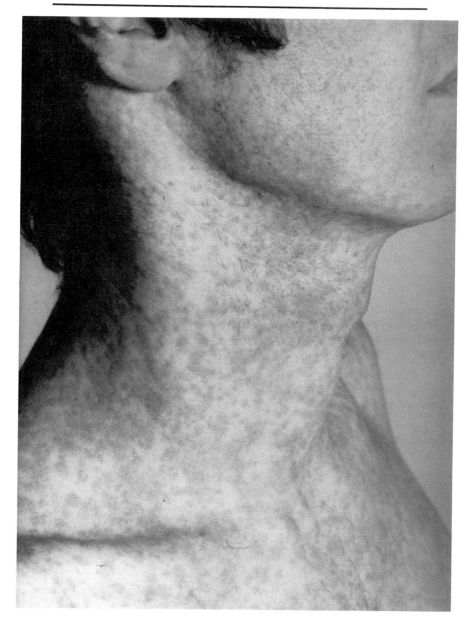

Mono brings with it many possible symptoms. A German measles-like rash, such as this, occurs in about 10 percent of mono patients.

mono. But their symptoms are not the typical symptoms that develop in adolescents.

The elderly may not have swollen lymph nodes, sore throat, or even atypical lymphocytes in blood samples. But fever almost always occurs. Fever may last longer than in younger patients—an average of thirteen days, compared to seven days in young adults. Elderly mono patients are also likely to suffer from tiredness and abdominal pain.

Our immune systems keep viruses in check. When the immune system of a person carrying EBV is weakened, the virus may reproduce more. The body in turn responds by

SYMPTOMS IN RELATION TO AGE[17]

Sign/Symptom	Patients under age 35	Patients over age 40
fever	89 %	95 %
sore throat	78 %	43 %
swollen lymph nodes	94 %	47 %
enlarged spleen	49 %	33 %
enlarged liver	6 %	42 %
jaundice	4 %	27 %
rash	7 %	12 %

producing more Epstein-Barr virus protein antibodies. Many studies have shown that older people have higher levels of Epstein-Barr virus antibodies, possibly because their immune systems are not able to handle the virus as well. But no link has been found between this increase in antibody production and any clinical consequences.[18]

4

Diagnosing Mono

Evelyn, a twenty-three-year-old receptionist, felt like she had a bad cold or flu. The doctor examined her and, suspecting mono, did a mono test. But the test was negative, so the doctor said it was probably just a cold and would go away on its own.

Evelyn felt exhausted, but she made herself go to work over the next week. Her neck was swollen, and she couldn't eat. Her throat got so sore she decided to go back to the doctor. After examining her throat, the doctor ran another blood test. This time it was positive—Evelyn had mono after all.[1]

Diagnosing Mono

When a teen or young adult comes to a doctor complaining of flulike symptoms, the possibility of mono may come to mind, because this is the age when mono usually occurs. The doctor will ask about symptoms and then examine the patients. He or she will take the patient's temperature, check the throat, feel the lymph nodes in the neck area, and feel the stomach area to see if the liver or spleen is enlarged.

But mono symptoms, especially in the beginning, can be misleading. The sore throat is sometimes mistaken for a strep throat infection. (The tonsils may become enlarged and covered with pus as happens in strep throat.) But strep can be ruled out if a throat culture—taken by wiping a cotton swab over the patient's throat and transferring the material it has picked up to a dish with culture medium—does not grow strep bacteria into visible colonies. A painful neck could be mistaken for a symptom of meningitis, a serious infection of the membranes that cover the brain or spinal cord. Abdominal pains might bring to mind acute appendicitis. Cough and throat lesions occur in diphtheria (a serious, formerly common childhood disease that is now prevented with the DPT vaccine); the rash is similar to that of rubella or measles; and swollen lymph glands are seen in AIDS and in some types of cancer.

Blood Tests

If the doctor suspects mono at all, some blood tests will be done. The first is a quick, inexpensive test based on the first definitive test for mono, developed back in 1932. It is called the Monospot test (spot test or heterophile antibody test). This test can often be done right in the doctor's office, with

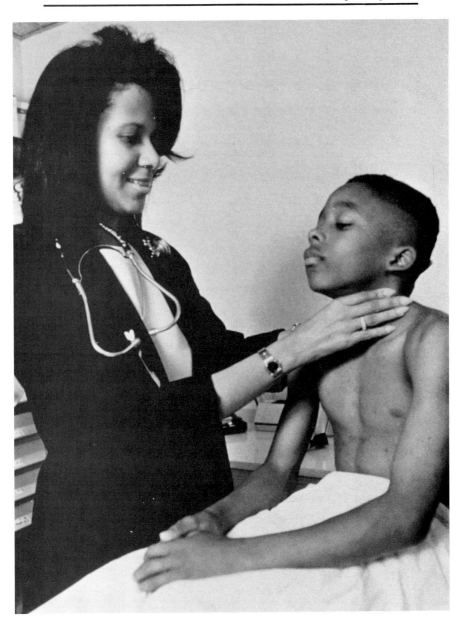

Doctors use many methods to diagnose mono. One of the first symptoms they check is whether the lymph nodes in the neck are swollen.

results in as little as three minutes. The spot test checks for heterophile antibodies (also called Paul-Bunnell antibodies, after the researchers who discovered the reaction), which can be detected in about 80 percent of mono patients.

A sample of the patient's blood is placed on a card that has been coated with dried material including red blood cells from a sheep or horse. The test is positive if the red blood cells clump together. The presence of these antibodies is an indication that the body is actively fighting the Epstein-Barr virus, but the level of heterophile antibodies in the blood is not related to how serious the symptoms are.

The Monospot test is usually accurate, but it can give false negative and false positive results. (Heterophile antibodies may remain in the blood for months, so a positive test does not necessarily mean current infection.) However, when a positive test is combined with the observation of symptoms, the doctor can usually make a diagnosis.

Sometimes when the test is negative but observable symptoms seem to point to mononucleosis, the test may be repeated after a week, since antibodies may not have appeared yet. Most people develop antibodies within the first week after symptoms have appeared. But in about 15 percent of cases the heterophile antibodies do not appear until after the first week.[2] Very young children may not show heterophile antibodies when they come down with infectious mononucleosis. Those with EBV infections that do not resemble classic mono are less likely to develop heterophile antibodies, too.

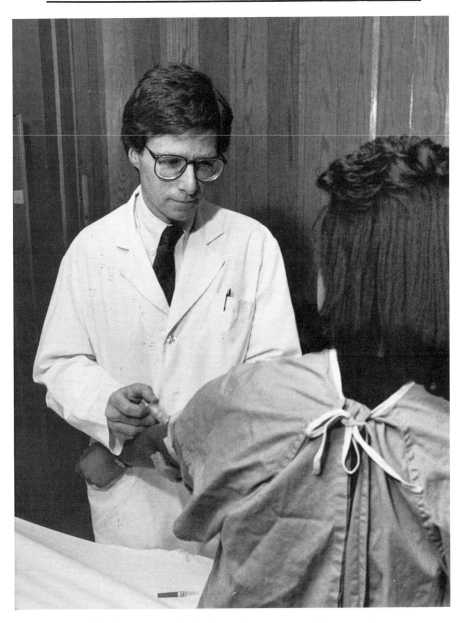

Blood tests are typically done whenever mono is suspected.

If the doctor's office has a laboratory, test results will be available during the visit. If not, then the patient will know within one or two days.

Another blood test, called a complete blood count (CBC), might also be used. It measures the number of red and white blood cells. The doctor will be looking for an increase in the number of white blood cells. Having 50 percent or more lymphocytes is an indication of mono. The blood sample may also be examined under the microscope to identify the classic atypical mononuclear lymphocytes, characteristic of mono.

If the results of the spot test are uncertain, a series of blood tests called an EBV serologic profile will give a definite diagnosis. These tests check for specific EBV antibodies. (Different antibodies are detectable at different stages of the illness.) The tests are highly accurate, but very expensive.

Special Considerations for the Elderly

A seventy-year-old woman went to the hospital with fever, sore throat, back pain, and dehydration. She had pain in her lower back after playing tennis, then developed fever, sore throat, headache, and nausea. A month before, she had visited a relative infected with mono. The slide test for heterophile antibodies was positive, but at first the numbers of lymphocytes and atypical lymphocytes were not high. Two weeks later, when she was readmitted to the hospital, these levels were higher.[3]

This woman was lucky that she thought of mentioning her exposure to mononucleosis and thus set her doctor

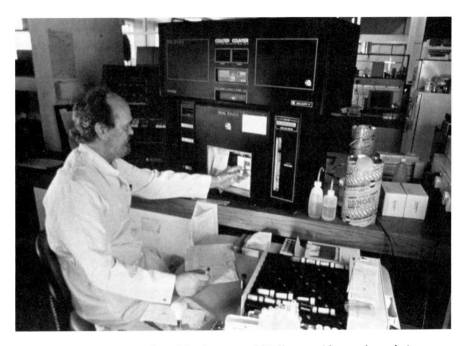

Sometimes a complete blood count (CBC) test (shown here being performed in a laboratory) is used to diagnose mono. The test measures the number of white and red blood cells in a given blood sample.

thinking along the right lines. Ordinarily, mono would not be one of a doctor's early guesses when dealing with an older patient. This disease is not very common in older age groups, and its symptoms in the elderly are not "typical" infectious mononucleosis symptoms. Numerous other diseases and illnesses might seem more likely to be the cause of the problem. For this reason, people over fifty-five are often subjected to a variety of tests to explore the other possibilities. Blood or urine tests for hepatitis or other infectious diseases may be run. X rays may be taken to rule out tuberculosis. Atypical lymphocytes can make the doctor suspect leukemia. Biopsies may be taken from lymph nodes or even the bone marrow because the doctor might think the patient has cancer. Many older people are diagnosed with "fever of unknown origin." Some of these patients may actually have infectious mononucleosis.[4]

Is Diagnosing Mono Worth the Bother?

Usually, a doctor's aim in running diagnostic tests is to find out specifically what is wrong with the patient so that the illness can be treated more effectively. But, as we'll see in the next chapter, there is not much that can be done for a mono patient. There are ways of easing some of the symptoms, but the body's own defenses have to bring the virus invasion under control. So, why bother going through the trouble and expense of laboratory tests to establish that a patient really does have infectious mononucleosis?

The main reason is that the symptoms of mono can also

be symptoms of other, much more serious diseases. Discovering that the problem is "only mono" can help to calm the patient's fears and also avoid having to run a lot of other tests for the more serious conditions. In addition, the patient can be advised what precautions to take to avoid making things worse. And the doctor will know what to watch for in case some of the rare, dangerous complications develop.

Recent news on the health care front has helped to put the value of diagnostic tests for mono into perspective. In 1993, the state of Oregon drew up a program extending medical coverage to all poor people but (to keep costs reasonable) limiting the services that would be provided under the plan. About 700 medical procedures were ranked according to their effectiveness, on the basis of consulting experts' opinions. Only the first 568 procedures would be covered. Treatment of common colds and infectious mononucleosis didn't make the cut and would not be covered, but the *diagnosis* of mononucleosis would be paid for under the Oregon program.[5]

5
Treating and Preventing Mononucleosis

Doctor, I feel like I'm dying," twenty-year-old Mary
Pierce told Dr. Halberstam over the phone.

"What exactly is wrong?" the doctor inquired.

"Everything," Mary replied. "My head hurts, my joints
hurt, I'm hot all over, my stomach aches, I can't swallow, I'm
so weak that I can barely move."

Dr. Halberstam told her to come in to his office. When
he examined her, he found she had a temperature of 102
degrees and swollen, tender lymph nodes; and her tonsils were
covered with a thick, whitish coating. The doctor told Mary
he was going to give her a blood test, but he was "99 percent
sure" she had mono.

"But doctor, I can't have mono. I've got a term paper to
finish next month, and I'm supposed to be married in June,
and I can't be sick that long."

The doctor assured her that she would probably be better in another two or three weeks, but unfortunately there wasn't anything he could give her to make the illness go away any faster.[1] That was back in 1974, only a few years after doctors had discovered that mononucleosis is caused by the Epstein-Barr virus. However, today the story is pretty much the same—doctors still have no cure for infectious mononucleosis.

For many illnesses doctors have medications that help the patient to recover more quickly and completely. But viral infections can't be cured with antibiotics, and the few antivirals that have been developed are not effective against EBV. So, other than suggesting that the patient get plenty of rest, drink plenty of fluids to prevent dehydration, and eat a well-balanced diet, doctors don't have much to offer the mono patient.

What to Do for a Mono Patient

Many doctors recommend that people with mono should stay home from school or work until all symptoms are gone and their energy level is back to normal.

College students away from home are sometimes hospitalized because they are often too weak to take care of themselves. But most people just stay in bed at home. The standard treatment used to be bed rest for four to six weeks, with limited activity for three months after all the symptoms were gone. Today, doctors recommend bed rest for one to three weeks, depending on how the patient feels, and avoiding strenuous exercise until recovery is complete.

Most patients recover on their own without any problems within four to six weeks from the time symptoms began. Symptoms may last longer in some patients, though. And some people believe that if you don't take it easy during the first two weeks of the illness, you could take much longer to recover.

Students often feel obligated to get back into their studies as soon as they can. Workers might worry about losing pay—or even losing their jobs—if they stay out sick too long. But when people insist on forcing themselves to meet a deadline or take a test when they should be resting, they run the risk of suffering a relapse and ending up back in bed. (Remember that stress can lower the body's defenses against EBV.)

Relieving Symptoms

Saltwater gargles are recommended for sore throats. Pain relievers such as acetaminophen are often recommended for headache and muscle pains. Most physicians advise against taking aspirin, however. In rare instances taking aspirin during viral diseases such as mono has been linked with a serious and often fatal illness called Reye's syndrome.

Special Precautions

Doctors often advise that activities should be limited by how the person feels. But, since half of mono patients suffer from

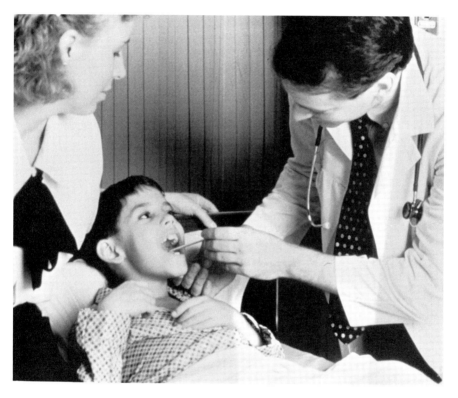

Sore throats are often a symptom of mono. Doctors recommend saltwater gargles to help ease the pain.

enlarged spleens, special care should be taken to prevent injury. (A hard blow to the spleen can cause it to rupture, resulting in life-threatening internal bleeding.) Competitive sports, lifting, and straining should be avoided until recovery is complete. So, even though mono patients who have enlarged spleens often feel better before the spleen has returned to normal, it is important not to do strenuous activity until the doctor has confirmed that it has returned to normal.

Treating Complications of Mono

Prednisone and other corticosteroid hormones are sometimes used to counter severe complications (which are extremely rare), such as encephalitis (an inflammation of the brain), thrombocytopenia (a lack of blood components called platelets that help in blood clotting), hemolytic anemia (a massive destruction of red blood cells), or blockage of the respiratory air passages.[2] These drugs are effective for mono complications because they act specifically on the killer T cells, whose response to the infected B cells is the cause of the inflammation. (Respiratory blockage responds best to this type of treatment.)[3] But corticosteroids are drugs with many powerful side effects. In addition to reducing swelling dramatically, they can also suppress the immune system, leaving a patient more susceptible to other infections. Corticosteroids are thus not used for uncomplicated mono cases.

Some people with mono develop secondary infections caused by bacteria, such as strep throat, and may need to be given antibiotics such as penicillin or erythromycin. One form

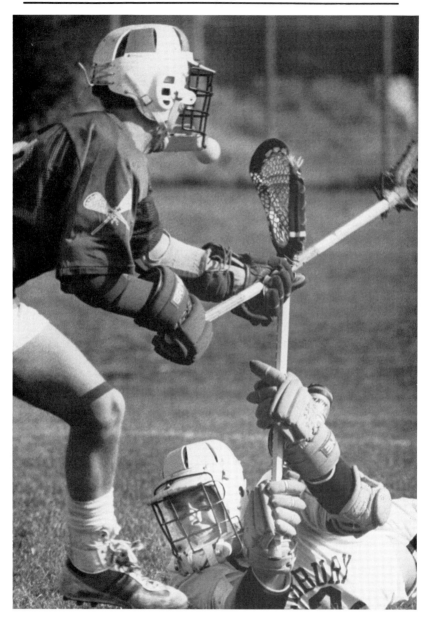

Competitive sports, such as lacrosse, should be avoided until recovery from mono is complete.

of penicillin, ampicillin, is not used—from 70 percent to 80 percent of mono patients given ampicillin develop a rash, although doctors don't know why.[4]

Preventing Mono

Doctors are always stressing the importance of taking precautions to prevent diseases before they happen. But so far researchers haven't turned up any good ideas about how to prevent infectious mononucleosis.

Eating well, getting plenty of exercise and rest, and reducing stress are known to help keep our immune systems strong, which keeps us healthier. However, researchers haven't been successful with immune-boosting strategies such as injections of gamma globulin (a fraction of blood serum that contains antibodies), for example.

Usually, we know that to avoid contact with a particular disease we should just stay away from people who have it until they are better. Unfortunately, with the Epstein-Barr virus, people may be contagious throughout their lives. The only real way to avoid mono would be to avoid kissing or close contact with anyone! Nobody, especially most teens and young adults, would think that sounds like a very good idea.

Special precautions are needed to protect people with defective immune systems from infection by EBV, however. Children with hereditary immune deficiencies, people with AIDS, and transplant recipients who are taking immune-suppressing drugs need to be especially careful. They could develop cancer from an EBV infection. Blood for transfusions and organs for transplants must be carefully tested or treated to eliminate viruses if they are to be used for immune-deficient people.

But in ordinary life, and even in a hospital, in most cases it is not necessary to isolate people suffering from mononucleosis. Commonsense precautions, such as washing one's hands after contact with patients or their body fluids, are usually good enough.[5]

Actually, some doctors say that it is probably not a good idea even to try to protect children from infection with Epstein-Barr virus, since that would just lead to their catching it at a later age, when they are more likely to have mono symptoms.[6] In fact, one way to avoid getting mono is to be infected with EBV while you are a child. But it is probably not a wise idea to deliberately expose children to the virus, since there is a small chance that they might develop serious—even life-threatening—complications.

In the future, a vaccine against the Epstein-Barr virus may be available. It would be given to young children to protect them from mononucleosis, without the risk of causing a more serious problem.

6

The Many Faces of EBV

Nine-year-old Michael was having trouble breathing. For a week he had been complaining of a sore throat and pain when he tried to swallow. His family doctor had prescribed penicillin, but the symptoms just got worse, and he was still running a fever. His tonsils were enlarged and infected, and his nose and throat were filled with bad-smelling secretions. His worried parents brought him to the hospital. Because Michael's condition was so serious, he was hospitalized for several weeks. Doctors ran several tests to determine what was causing the boy's symptoms. A mono test was positive. Michael was given steroid drugs to help reduce the blockage. For several days he was still very sick, and he became confused and upset. He made a harsh rasping noise with each breath. But by the fifth day in the hospital he was much better, and a week later he was well enough to go home.[1]

Complications of Infectious Mononucleosis

Most people recover from mono without any problems—nine out of ten people with mono have no complications, although fatigue and weakness often persist for a month or more. Adults over thirty often have more severe and longer lasting symptoms.

Mono sometimes, although very rarely (in only one out of every three thousand cases[2]), causes death from complications such as inflammation of the heart (myocarditis) or the

TROUBLE BREATHING

Severe upper airway blockage is one of the most alarming complications of mononucleosis. Swollen tissues may completely fill the nasal passages, so that the person cannot breathe in enough oxygen. This complication occurs most often in younger patients, typically just before they reach puberty, and somewhat more often in boys than in girls. In one study, the average age for mono patients with severe difficulty in breathing was only eleven years old—much lower than the average of seventeen to twenty-five for most mono patients. A similar degree of respiratory blockage has more effect on younger patients because their airways are narrower.[3]

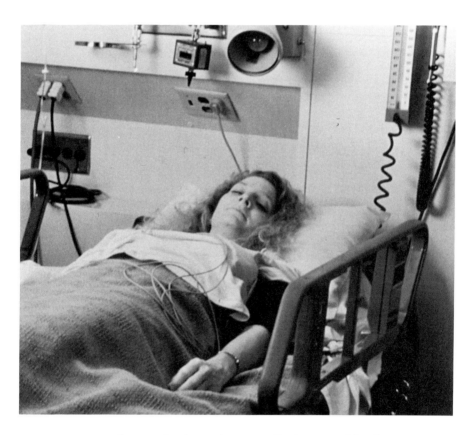

Rare cases of mono develop serious complications, requiring long-term treatment in the hospital.

membranes covering it (pericarditis), pneumonia, liver problems, and airway obstruction (the tonsils or other tissue may become so enlarged that the airways are blocked, making it difficult to breathe).

Steroid drugs are used to treat some of these complications. Airway obstruction sometimes requires an emergency operation. A temporary opening in the throat, called a tracheostomy, is made so that the patient can breathe.

Rupture of the spleen is another potentially life-threatening mono complication. The spleen filters the blood, removing bacteria, worn-out red blood cells, and bits of dead matter. Disease-fighting white blood cells congregate there, just as in the lymph nodes. (That is why the spleen typically becomes enlarged during mono—it has become a major battlefield in the body's fight against EBV.) Enlargement puts a strain on the spleen's spongy structure. If it tears open—from a sudden blow or on its own—blood spills out from the spleen's reservoirs into the body cavity. Large blood transfusions will be needed, and the organ will have to be surgically removed.

Less than one percent of mono cases involve neurological complications such as meningitis (inflammation of the membranes covering the brain or spinal cord) or encephalitis (inflammation of the brain tissue itself). These complications can cause seizures, convulsions, or even death.

In very rare instances, some people with mono suffer from a form of paralysis, resulting from involvement of the spinal cord, that is called the Guillain-Barré syndrome. In this condition the muscles of the legs and arms become weak and sometimes temporarily paralyzed. This complication usually goes away by itself, but sufferers may be weakened for weeks or months. Doctors don't have any treatment for this rare complication.

EBV and Cancer

Mononucleosis has been called "a self-limited leukemia" because it is like leukemia in some ways. In both diseases, white blood cells reproduce in large numbers. The body is able to get mono but not cancer under control. Mono only resembles cancer, but EBV infection can sometimes lead to cancer. (EBV is one of only four viruses ever shown without doubt to be associated with cancer.) Several types of cancer are suspected to be linked with EBV, including Burkitt's lymphoma, nasopharyngeal carcinoma, and Hodgkin's disease.

Burkitt's Lymphoma

As discussed in Chapter 2, Burkitt's lymphoma is a tumor of the jaw that occurs most often in children who live in hot or humid regions of Africa. In girls, tumors sometimes occur in the ovaries. The tumors usually spread quickly through the body, resulting in death. Children with long and heavy exposure to EBV are at increased risk of developing Burkitt's lymphoma.[4] Practically all cases occur in areas of Africa where malaria is widespread. Scientists believe malaria's effect on the body's disease-fighting system could cause an abnormal response to infection with Epstein-Barr virus. Then, instead

60

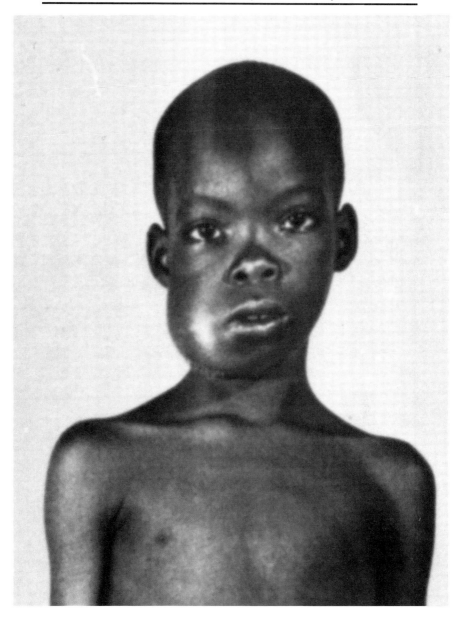

This child has Burkitt's lymphoma, a tumor of the jaw that occurs most often in children who live in Africa.

of causing excess lymphocytes to be produced, as occurs in infectious mononucleosis, EBV causes lymphoid tissue to become cancerous.[5]

Recently, scientists have concluded that EBV is only a cofactor in Burkitt's lymphoma, rather than the main cause. Some patients suffering from the cancer are not infected with EBV. Researchers believe that the lymphoma develops when the chromosomes become rearranged or mixed up in B lymphocytes. The Epstein-Barr virus contributes by greatly increasing the number of B lymphocytes, and thus increasing the chances for the mix-up to occur. But the virus isn't necessary.[6]

Some researchers believe that the milk bush, a plant commonly used to treat various diseases in areas where Burkitt's lymphoma is found, may be involved in the disease. In laboratory studies, researchers have found that extracts from the plant magnify the effects of EBV on human chromosomes, particularly chromosome 8. This chromosome activates a gene that can cause malignant changes in lymphocytes that have previously been infected with EBV. Laboratory experiments exposing B lymphocytes to the active ingredient in the milk bush plant and to EBV, led to a rearrangement of the chromosomes. This chromosome rearrangement was not found when the white blood cells were exposed to the milk bush plant extract or EBV separately.[7]

Nasopharyngeal Carcinoma

Nasopharyngeal carcinoma is a cancer of the nose and throat that affects up to 80,000 people each year.[8] It is particularly common among the Southern Chinese and Chinese who have immigrated to Malaysia and Singapore. In southern China, at least 25 percent of all cancers are nasopharyngeal carcinomas. This form of cancer is also common among Eskimos. It is the number-one tumor affecting Eskimo men and the second most common for Eskimo women.[9] Epstein-Barr virus is always found in the tumors. EBV does not cause the disease by itself, since nearly all of the world is infected with EBV and most people do not get this disease. But it is apparently a major factor.

Hodgkin's Disease

In March 1993, National Hockey League star Mario Lemieux was able to rejoin his Pittsburgh Penguins teammates two months after he received eight weeks of radiation treatment for a form of lymph cancer called Hodgkin's disease. Also called Hodgkin's lymphoma, the disease was named after a nineteenth-century English physician, Thomas Hodgkin. The cause of Hodgkin's disease is unknown, but many different infections are suspected, including viruses such as the Epstein-Barr virus.

Hodgkin's disease (HD) is a painless swelling of the lymph nodes in the neck, armpits, or groin, accompanied by tiredness, weakness, loss of appetite, weight loss, fever, night sweats, itching, and anemia. It is fairly rare, with between 5,000 and 6,000 new cases diagnosed each year in the United States. It is more common in young people from fifteen to thirty-five years of age; it may also occur in people between fifty-five and seventy. Curiously, it tends to strike mainly people from an educated well-to-do background, and many patients are only children or have few brothers or sisters.

The swollen lymph nodes typical of Hodgkin's disease are due to runaway reproduction by cells in the lymph nodes. These cells, called Reed-Sternberg cells, have a characteristic appearance, which allows doctors to diagnose four different types of Hodgkin's lymphomas by looking at a tissue sample from an enlarged lymph node under a microscope.

Hodgkin's disease is treated with radiation therapy when it is detected early. From 80 percent to 90 percent of these patients recover completely. If the disease is not detected until it has spread to other organs in the body, it is treated with chemotherapy, using anticancer drugs. At this stage, treatment

PORTRAIT OF A HODGKIN'S SURVIVOR

Susan came home from Vietnam in 1971 after a grueling tour of duty as a military nurse. At twenty-four she had her life ahead of her. But she felt tired all the time, and physical activities—like hiking or dancing—left her gasping for breath. "I thought I was really, really out of shape," she says. But when she began coughing up blood, she knew her problem was more serious. Her doctor ordered X rays, which showed tumors in her chest. A biopsy of tissue samples confirmed a diagnosis of Hodgkin's disease. Radiation treatments brought a complete cure.[10]

is only 40 percent effective. However, in the past Hodgkin's disease was almost always fatal.

For years researchers have suspected that this disease is linked with EBV because an increased level of EBV antibodies has been found in some Hodgkin's disease patients; also, tissues taken from some patients contained EBV DNA. Moreover, people who develop mono have an increased risk of developing HD.[11] In one study of nearly ten thousand mononucleosis patients, seven developed Hodgkin's disease—that is, about four times the expected number. Most of these cases occurred among females within three years of their developing mono.[12] Some studies have found that 35 percent of cases of Hodgkin's disease may be associated with EBV.[13] There is also a suggestive similarity in the patterns of cases of Hodgkin's disease and mono—both occur mainly among young people who were less likely to have been exposed to common disease germs as children.

However, many researchers do not believe EBV is a cause of Hodgkin's disease. First of all, not all HD patients have EBV antibodies. Moreover, both mono and HD occur in higher socioeconomic groups. People who develop both diseases have lowered immunities and are thus more susceptible. Researchers point out that association is "weak at best."[14]

Can EBV Make People More Susceptible to Cancers in General?

Since EBV is involved with nasopharyngeal carcinoma and Burkitt's lymphoma, some may wonder whether EBV can make a person more susceptible to cancers in general, later in life. Most researchers do not believe so. But, in one study, researchers found that healthy members of families with multiple cases of cancer had higher EBV antibody levels than normal. The researchers suggested that high EBV antibody levels may be a sign that members of the family have abnormal immune systems and may be susceptible to cancer.[15]

Sjögren's Syndrome

The Epstein-Barr virus may also be involved in Sjögren's syndrome, a chronic autoimmune disease in which the body attacks its own tissues. In this syndrome, severe dryness of the eyes and mouth result from destruction of salivary and lacrimal (tear) glands. One explanation for the body's attack against these glands might be that EBV infection of the salivary glands sensitizes the body's defenders not only to infected cells but also to other glandular cells. Researchers aren't sure whether EBV reactivation causes the immune system to go wrong, or whether the EBV reactivates after the immune system has already gone wrong.[16]

Why Does EBV Cause Mono in Some People and Cancer in Others?

Why does the Epstein-Barr virus cause cancer in some people and mild symptoms of mononucleosis in others? Researchers believe that something else is required to trigger the cancer. Many believe the trigger is something that weakens the immune system.

In 1984 this idea was confirmed when doctors learned a little more about EBV from a tragic case. David, a real boy in Texas whose condition was the basis for the 1976 movie *The Boy in the Plastic Bubble,* died after undergoing an operation that was meant to help him live a normal life. Like two hundred other children born each year, David had severe combined immunodeficiency (SCID). Normal bone marrow produces a number of blood cells, including the B and T lymphocytes. But these cells are not produced in people with SCID. Without these disease-fighting cells, David couldn't fight off the simplest infection. Even a cold could kill him.

After David was born in 1972, his family and doctors decided to keep him alive in a special plastic bubble to keep out all germs until a cure could be found. In 1984 he received a bone marrow transplant from his sister. Doctors hoped he would be able to produce immune-defending white blood cells on his own after the operation. But four months later David died of cancer. Hiding in his sister's bone marrow was the Epstein-Barr virus. It can live in our bodies and never bother us, because our immune defenses keep it in check. But David had no immune defenses. The B cells that he had received through the bone marrow transplant went out of control. He died of a cancer that resembles Burkitt's lymphoma.[17]

Today, before bone marrow transplants are performed, doctors check the donor for Epstein-Barr virus and many other infectious agents that don't cause problems in healthy people. Improvements in the transplant operation and better drug treatments have helped make it possible for children with immune problems to live without spending their lives in a plastic bubble.[18]

The theory that a weakened immune system plays an important role has also been reinforced by observations of AIDS patients, whose immune systems are damaged. These patients often develop mouth sores called hairy leukoplakia after being infected with or reactivating EBV. EBV infection can also lead to lymphomas in transplant patients who are taking immune-suppressing drugs to keep their bodies from rejecting the new donor organs.

In the case of Burkitt's lymphoma, doctors believe malaria paves the way for cancer by compromising the immune system. It's like cigarette smoking and lung cancer. Very heavy and early exposure to EBV is as though you were smoking two packs of cigarettes per day all your life. Then malaria depresses part of the immune system that helps to control B cells. And then something transforms B cells into tumor cells.

Heredity may also play an important role. Children with a rare genetic disorder called Purtilo's syndrome (also known as Duncan's syndrome, or X-linked lymphoproliferative syndrome) are defenseless against EBV infection and almost always develop fatal complications when exposed to EBV. The "X-linked" variation of the name for the disorder means that the gene responsible for it is found on one of the chromosomes containing the instructions for sex characteristics, and the disorder occurs only in boys.

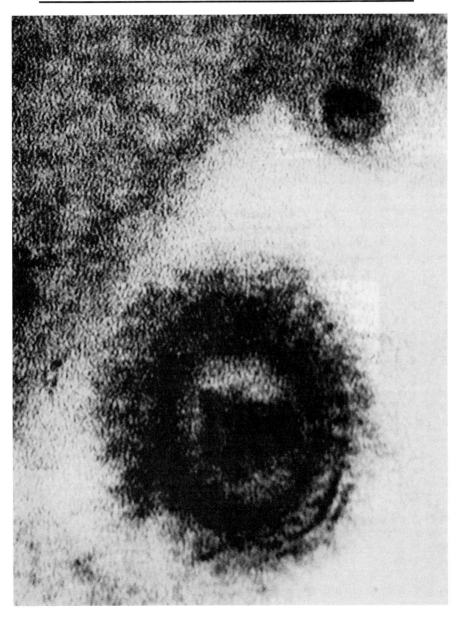

An electron micrograph of the Epstein-Barr virus. Doctors now routinely check for the presence of this virus before performing bone marrow transplants.

How Can EBV Be Involved in So Many Different Diseases?

A weakened immune system may explain how EBV can cause disease in people, but it doesn't explain why it may cause so many different types of disease. Part of the reason may depend on what type of tissue the virus infects. The first symptoms of mono include a sore throat while the virus is reproducing in epithelial cells in the throat lining. Further symptoms of mono are caused by the body's response to infected B lymphocytes. Various lymphomas develop when infected B cells that were kept under control by the body suddenly begin reproducing wildly. Hairy leukoplakia is an infection of the surface of the tongue with several strains of EBV, characterized by explosive, although localized, viral replication.[20]

How can we explain the fact that almost everyone is infected with EBV but there are very few cases of clinically apparent disease? Researchers at St. Jude Children's Hospital in Memphis, Tennessee, believe that some Epstein-Barr viruses may be responsible for causing disease, whereas other EBV strains produce no symptoms. For years doctors have known that there are two groups of EBV: EBV type A and type B (also called EBV-1 and EBV-2). Researchers have also found other important differences among EBV viruses. For example, EBV taken from fresh throat washings infected epithelial cells in the laboratory much more easily than the viruses grown in lymphocytes.

7

Chronic Fatigue Syndrome

I n 1985 the news was filled with stories about a strange new illness. It all began when Paul Cheney and Daniel Peterson, two doctors in Incline Village, Nevada (a small resort town in the Lake Tahoe area), reported that a number of their patients were suffering from a mysterious fatigue that had lasted for months and months. Many of these patients had sore throats, swollen lymph nodes, and swollen spleens or livers. Since the symptoms were similar to those of mononucleosis, the doctors labeled the condition "chronic Epstein-Barr infection" or "chronic mononucleosis."

News about the Nevada doctors' findings spread quickly. Similar clusters of cases were found around the nation. One third of the faculty of a high school came down with chronic Epstein-Barr infection. An entire girl's basketball team was sidelined with the strange illness.[1] Many of the patients were middle-class professionals, and the media quickly named the mysterious illness "yuppie flu" or "yuppie plague." The strange new illness seemed to affect women more than men. The exhaustion was so bad that one woman said she felt like Raggedy Ann without the stuffing. The media then came up with another name for the illness: the "Raggedy Ann syndrome." *Newsweek* magazine called it "the malaise of the eighties."

Major studies about chronic Epstein-Barr infection appeared in *Science* magazine, *The New York Times,* and *Rolling Stone,* and it was even featured on ABC TV's *20/20.* One researcher suggested that twelve million Americans would come down with the disease in the next few years. Some said the estimate was too high, but probably tens of thousands would be involved. People of all ages and all walks of life would be vulnerable, not just "yuppies." In fact, investigators for the Centers for Disease Control (CDC) found that patients already diagnosed with the illness ranged from eight to more than seventy years old.[2]

Chronic Mononucleosis?

This was not the first time there had been reports of a chronic disease with symptoms resembling those of infectious mononucleosis. In fact, there had been numerous reports of "chronic mononucleosis" in medical journals, dating back for decades. But they had not received attention in the popular press, and many doctors were skeptical about the idea that they were really mono.

It was not really unreasonable to believe that EBV could cause a chronic disease. Nearly everyone on Earth is eventually infected with the Epstein-Barr virus. And by the time the "yuppie flu" stories hit the headlines, it had already been shown that once a person is infected with EBV, the virus remains in the body, even though there are no longer any symptoms of illness. Perhaps in some individuals the immune system is not able to keep the virus in check, and the continuous battle inside the body causes the chronic fatigue and monolike symptoms. Critics, however, pointed out that if EBV caused long-lasting fatigue, civilization would never have made it this far because the virus affects almost everyone.

Scientists from the Centers for Disease Control were sent out to investigate the clusters of illness. They found that the symptoms were real, but found no evidence to link EBV to the illness. The CDC team concluded that chronic EBV disease and chronic mononucleosis were not appropriate descriptions. The team suggested the name should be changed to chronic mononucleosis-like syndrome. (A syndrome is a group of symptoms that tend to occur together.) Eventually the condition was renamed chronic fatigue syndrome (CFS).

Defining Chronic Fatigue System

In 1988 the CDC made a case definition for the ailment. To be diagnosed with chronic fatigue syndrome, victims must have debilitating fatigue lasting six months or more, with activity reduced by 50 percent. No other disease can be present that might bring on similar symptoms, including cancer, autoimmune ailments, or AIDS, or any preexisting psychiatric disease. Patients must also exhibit most of the following symptoms: headache, fever, sore throat, muscle aches, joint pain, generalized muscle weakness, lymph node pain, prolonged fatigue following exercise, sleep problems, confusion and forgetfulness, and visual problems; and symptoms must have developed suddenly over a few hours or days.[3] There is no mention of EBV in the official CDC definition.

TEEN TURMOIL

Eleven-year-old Hoben Spalding and his single mother, Chris Spalding, came down with an intestinal virus, from which they couldn't seem to recover. Chris Spalding says, "Hoben would fall asleep twenty times a night doing his homework, or he would fall asleep over an open drawer, looking for a T shirt. Once he even fell asleep petting our dog." Truant officers stopped by to lecture Hoben when he was home sick, and his teachers thanked him sarcastically when he came to class. "When he was twelve, Hoben talked about suicide. Eventually Hoben was allowed to attend eighth grade for half-days, but "they still believe it's an attitude, not an illness."[4]

Taking CFS Seriously

Forty-one-year-old Sharon Dieppa was so tired she couldn't go to work. She underwent numerous tests to rule out various causes, but they didn't find anything. She believed she had CFS. But her doctor said, "I'm sorry, but I don't believe in that illness."[5] That was a common reaction in the 1980s. Now doctors are more likely to accept a diagnosis of CFS. A study at the end of 1991, for example, found that 71 percent of physicians accepted the existence of chronic fatigue syndrome.[6]

Searching for a Cause

Today most health experts recognize chronic fatigue syndrome as a real ailment, but no one is yet sure what the cause is. Since EBV was first suspected, researchers have found evidence linking other viruses to CFS. Some researchers, such as Dr. Anthony L. Komaroff of the Brigham and Women's Hospital in Boston, believe a newly discovered herpesvirus, HHV-6 (human herpesvirus number six), might be involved. It attacks white blood cells of the immune system. Unlike EBV, however, it also attacks other immune cells and nervous-system cells too. It is also an extremely widespread virus, like EBV.

Recently, still another virus has been found in the white blood cells of CFS sufferers. Dr. Elaine DeFreitas at the Wistar Institute in Philadelphia has found evidence linking CFS to a retrovirus similar to a retrovirus called HTLV-II, which causes hairy cell leukemia (a rare blood cancer). John

Martin, chief of immunopathology at the University of Southern California, believes a different retrovirus, called a spuma virus or foamy virus, is involved. (HIV-1 and HIV-2—the viruses that cause AIDS—are the only other retroviruses found in humans besides the HTLV and human foamy viruses.)

Peter Behan of the University of Glasgow, Scotland, is studying the possibility of a link of CFS with enteroviruses (the class of viruses that includes the polio virus.)

"Several infectious agents may be playing a role here," says Dr. Robert Schooley, chief of the infectious diseases section at the University of Colorado Health Sciences Center in Denver.[7] Many researchers agree. Some say that several different viruses working together could actually interact to produce CFS. Walter J. Gunn, who heads CFS program activities at CDC in Atlanta, says there is some evidence that reactivation of a latent infection with EBV, HHV-6, or cytomegalovirus could bring on CFS-type symptoms. Other evidence shows that something is causing the immune system to be suppressed, which may point to a virus similar to HTLV-II. "A retrovirus can have effects on the immune system, and possibly the immune system could be allowing the reactivation of these latent herpesviruses," says Walter Gunn. "None of it is proven, but it is one model we're thinking of."[8]

An Immune System Problem

Researchers are finding increasing evidence that chronic fatigue syndrome is an immune system disorder, and many now call the illness CFIDS—chronic fatigue immune dysfunction syndrome. "The pattern that is emerging is a chronically activated immune system, an immune system engaged in some kind of chronic war against some kind of thing that it perceives as foreign," says Dr. Komaroff.[9]

Unlike AIDS, in which a virus causes the immune system to be suppressed, leaving infected individuals susceptible to infections, chronic fatigue syndrome patients have immune systems that are working too hard. This mysterious illness might begin when something—perhaps allergies, or a virus, or some other environmental factor—damages the immune system and enables viruses that are normally held in check to begin reproducing. Then the efforts of the immune system to defend the body could cause the symptoms of CFIDS.

Other Possible Explanations

Researchers are also finding other evidence to support the idea that chronic fatigue syndrome has a physical basis. CFS patients have definite neurological problems. They don't perform well on certain tests of thinking ability. Using sophisticated devices, other researchers have shown that CFS patients often show abnormally low blood flow to one of the two lobes of the brain. Dr. Anthony Komaroff at the Brigham and Women's Hospital in Boston has found evidence of brain inflammation in people suffering from CFS.[10]

Other researchers suspect that CFS may have something to do with a hormonal problem. Stephen E. Straus, chief of the laboratory of clinical investigation at the National

Institute of Allergy and Infectious Diseases and colleagues at the National Institute of Mental Health and the University of Michigan found that CFS patients have altered levels of certain brain hormones.[11]

Is There Any Treatment for CFS?

Doreen was a physician who enjoyed an active life. She ate a low-fat vegetarian diet, exercised regularly, and took good care of herself. Then, suddenly, she developed severe fatigue, which seemed to hang on for months. Her throat felt sore on and off, and she felt feverish. Sometimes she couldn't get up out of bed; she kept forgetting things and couldn't concentrate on her work. A thorough checkup didn't reveal anything except that she had high levels of antibodies to EBV, cytomegalovirus, and hepatitis virus in her blood. Doreen was diagnosed as having chronic fatigue syndrome. Over time the symptoms became less severe and less frequent.[12]

Other than recommending eating as best as you can, and getting plenty of rest and exercise, doctors don't have much to offer in the way of treatment for CFS. However, most CFS sufferers recover on their own. Many are bedridden for months before they get better. Others suffer for years, and some have not yet recovered. Doctors are experimenting with various treatments, including antidepressant drugs and special exercise programs. Some CFS sufferers have found relief with an experimental AIDS drug, Ampligen.[13] Among the 50 percent to 80 percent of CFS patients who have food allergies,

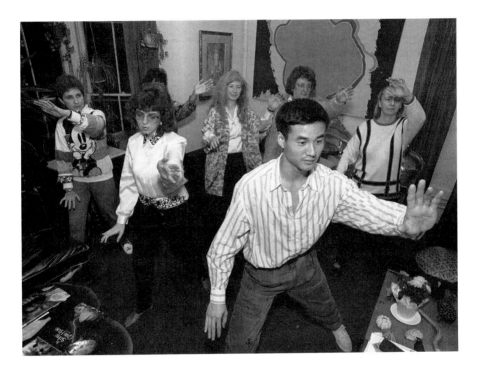

Doctors are experimenting with special exercise programs in the treatment of Chronic Fatigue Syndrome. Here, Joseph Cheu leads a group of CFS patients through Tai Chi.

avoiding the foods to which the are sensitive may help to eliminate CFS symptoms.[14]

The Disease of the Nineties

Scientists will eventually figure out whether or not the Epstein-Barr virus or the several other viruses that have been suspected are really linked to chronic fatigue immune dysfunction syndrome. And if they aren't, researchers will eventually discover what the cause or causes of this mysterious illness really are.

Walter J. Gunn, who heads CFS program activities at the Centers for Disease Control in Atlanta, says that our knowledge about CFS is similar to where our knowledge about AIDS was a decade ago, when scientists didn't know which of the many medical problems they were seeing was the cause of AIDS and which were just "opportunistic hangers-on."[15]

Meanwhile, CFS continues to plague thousands of people each year. Many experts think that CFS is being overdiagnosed—it is becoming a catch-all for many who are simply depressed or who suffer from other fatigue-related illnesses. Others say it is still greatly underdiagnosed. The Centers for Disease Control has set up surveillance studies in Atlanta, Georgia, in Reno, Nevada, in Grand Rapids, Michigan, and in Wichita, Kansas, to try to better understand the problem. In the early 1990s, the CDC received one to two thousand calls each month from people who thought they had chronic fatigue syndrome.[16] In 1991, the CDC estimated that there are at least 100,000 cases in the United States.[17]

Dr. Jay Levy predicts CFS will be the "disease of the nineties," as the public and the medical community become more aware of it.[18] By the early 1990s, there were already four national organizations and more than four hundred local support groups for those who suffer from this mysterious but debilitating illness.

8

The Future of Mononucleosis

Scientists have a lot of questions to answer before they completely understand how the Epstein-Barr virus can be involved in such a wide range of diseases. But a lot of progress is being made, and, as more is understood, they can better learn how to prevent the virus from causing harm.

An important discovery was how EBV causes the body to make extra B cells. In the late 1980s, Kevin Moore and Tim Mosmann of DNAX Research Institute in Palo Alto discovered an immune system regulator called IL-10 (interleukin-10) and cloned the gene containing the instructions for producing it. In a normal immune system, IL-10 increases the production of B lymphocytes and makes the T cells less active. The DNAX researchers discovered that EBV has a similar gene! "It's the ideal thing for this virus to have captured," says Moore.[1] EBV produces IL-10 to turn down the immune response against the virus, and at the same time causes the infected person to produce the B cells that it infects, giving it more targets to attack.

Another question that baffled researchers for some time was why the virus seemed to choose to infect B lymphocytes over other cell types. Many viruses can enter into a cell by attaching to special receptor sites on the cell surface. A specific molecule on the surface of the virus fits perfectly into the receptor site like a key in a lock. Scientists located the receptor for Epstein-Barr virus on B lymphocytes a number of years ago. It is called CR2 (also known as CD21). Scientists believe that a similar binding protein on epithelial cells and T cells explains why the virus can also infect those cells. The antigen

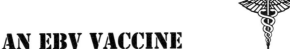

AN EBV VACCINE

Vaccines are usually developed for the purpose of preventing diseases. But an EBV vaccine could also serve as a valuable research tool. Scientists are still not sure about EBV's role in the many cancers it has been accused of being involved in. The only thing that is known for certain is that it is not the only cause. Vaccination for EBV, however, would remove a link in a chain of events that leads to these cancers and thus help clarify the role of this virus. Scientists hope to use a vaccine as proof that EBV is or is not involved in various diseases.

on the virus that fits into this receptor is called gp340. (The gp stands for glycoprotein, which is a combination of protein and sugar.) Scientists have also isolated other proteins that help the virus get into cells. The body builds up antibodies against these virus antigens that prevent the virus from attaching to the receptor sites.[2] Now scientists are using this information to try to develop a vaccination against Epstein-Barr virus infection. Dr. Michael Anthony Epstein, the co-discoverer of the virus, is one of the researchers working on an EBV vaccination.

Working Toward a Vaccination

Scientists have made a lot of progress toward developing an EBV vaccination. The gene that contains the instructions for the gp340 antigen was identified, and the sequence of the nucleic acid units in it was determined. For a human vaccine to be useful, scientists need large quantities of pure gp340. Researchers were able to clone the glycoprotein, by inserting its gene into bacteria, yeasts, and several types of mammalian cells. Dr. Andrew Morgan at the University of Bristol in England developed a technique that produces large amounts of purified gp340 from EBV-infected cells grown in the laboratory.

Dr. Epstein has tested a vaccine using gp340 on a species of cottontop tamarin monkeys. Dr. Epstein found that all of the monkeys that did not receive the vaccine developed lymphomas within a few weeks, but none of those that were vaccinated did. Dr. Epstein says "the vaccine is capable of protecting the animals against massive doses of tumor-inducing virus."[3] The gp340 vaccine also stimulated antibody production in mice and rabbits that were tested. However, at first, the antigen itself could not produce a strong enough immune response to protect humans.

Researchers are experimenting with several ideas for making the body's immune response greater. Dr. Epstein's group added a synthetic form of a natural body substance called threonyl muramyl dipeptide to the vaccine to increase the body's immune response. "We believe that this material is suitable for a first-generation vaccine to be used in man. This vaccine is safe and evokes a powerful humoral immune response as well as cellular immunity in the animal model," Dr. Epstein said.[4]

In the first tests of a vaccine using gp340, the virus was grown in cell cultures. However, this is not desirable because virus DNA can contaminate the vaccine, increasing the risk that vaccination could cause illness. The more purified gp340 that can now be produced using genetic engineering technology is referred to as recombinant gp340 because its gene was removed from the EBV virus and recombined with the genetic material of a bacterium or some other cell that can be conveniently grown in the laboratory. Recombinant gp340 has the advantage that it contains only the EBV glycoprotein and none of the EBV genes that could cause tumors. However, material produced from a recombinant source has to be rigorously tested before it can be approved by regulatory authorities.

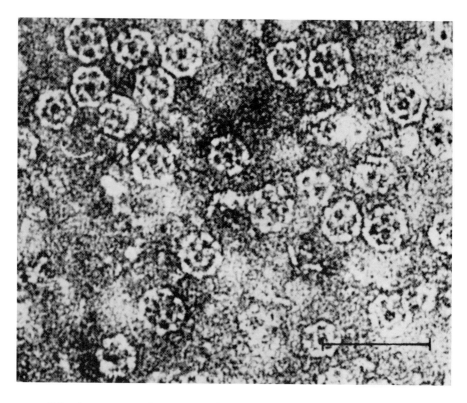

Scientists are experimenting with a vaccine using recombinant gp340 (shown here in an electron micrograph) to prevent mono.

Other Vaccine Possibilities

An alternative approach is to use recombinant technology to incorporate the gene that produces the virus antigens that the body recognizes, into a virus that doesn't cause harm in humans. Vaccinia virus, a specially attenuated (weakened) virus that was used to immunize people against smallpox, is now being used to carry many experimental vaccines, including EBV. Live viruses are likelier to produce a more broad-ranging and appropriate immune response, and would also be cheaper to produce. The disadvantage of using live viruses, however, is that there is a remote possibility that the harmless virus may gain back the ability to cause disease. There may also be more frequent side effects using live vaccinia.

 MONEY AND MEDICINE

Often the paths in medicine that are pursued are the ones where there will be a monetary payoff. This is because much medical research is funded by pharmaceutical companies, which cannot afford to invest in projects that will not be profitable. A vaccination for EBV is eagerly awaited because nearly 100,000 people die each year from Burkitt's lymphoma and nasopharyngeal cancer. But these diseases are common only in poorer developing nations. Some researchers are hopeful, however, that the link of EBV with some cases of Hodgkin's disease (which is much more common in the United States) will be an incentive to spend money in pursuit of an EBV vaccination.[6]

SEARCHING FOR AN ANIMAL MODEL

Vaccines that might be useful in saving human lives need to be tested on animals first, to show that they are safe to test on humans. But mice, rats, rabbits, and the other animals typically used in laboratory tests are not really suitable for testing EBV vaccines. They produce antibodies against the virus, but the antibodies can't be shown to protect them from disease—because the Epstein-Barr virus does not infect them in the first place.

Scientists have found very few animals that can be infected by EBV. So far, in fact, EBV infection has been observed only in monkeys. The common marmoset, for example, develops a monolike illness. In the early 1970s researchers discovered that some primates develop lymphomas after being injected with EBV. The cottontop tamarin develops malignant lymphomas at several sites within two to three weeks after the injection and ultimately dies. These tumors greatly resemble those that occur in human organ-transplant recipients. Because a very large dose of EBV must be used, any vaccine that could protect the tamarins from developing the tumors would probably be effective against the worst human infections. So the cottontop tamarin is thought to be a good model for testing vaccines against EBV.[5]

Furthermore, virus carriers are not yet suitable for EBV. In tests at the University of Bristol, three out of four tamarins injected with a stronger strain of recombinant vaccinia became immunized, but none injected with a weaker strain became immunized. "Should a live virus vaccinia vector become desirable, then it is clear that further work must be carried out to produce a virus which is sufficiently attenuated yet capable of inducing a suitably strong immune response," Dr. Andrew Morgan notes.[7]

Other viruses, such as modified forms of the adenovirus that causes colds, are also being used in vaccination experiments with tamarins. An adenovirus vaccine can be given orally, rather than by injection. This approach not only is more convenient but also may act directly on cells in the throat lining, increasing the protection against EBV infection.

Researchers in the University of Bristol experiment made a surprising observation. The three out of four tamarins that survived after being inoculated with EBV did not build up antibodies to gp340. The researchers concluded that a large part of the protective response of the body involves "cell-mediated immunity," in which T cells learn to recognize virus antigens and attack the virus directly.

Problems to Be Worked Out

People who develop nasopharyngeal carcinoma (NPC) do so later in life, long after being infected with EBV. Can a vaccine against EBV be used in people who have already been infected, to protect them from developing NPC later? That is one question that researchers are exploring.

Another question that is still unresolved is whether adding other EBV antigens would make the vaccine more effective. Researchers may have to incorporate other EBV glycoproteins such as gp85, which is involved in fusion of the virus with the host cell membrane, to produce a strong protective response.

Beginning Trials

Researchers have been hoping to begin trials in humans for some time. The first trials, involving young volunteers, will be designed to determine whether antibodies are built up and will also include a number of other immunological tests to see if the vaccine functions as it is supposed to. The vaccine will also be tested on children with Duncan's syndrome, who face a life-threatening situation if they are infected with EBV.

Phase II of the trials will focus on finding out whether college students who have not been infected with EBV will develop mononucleosis before they graduate. Dr. Epstein envisions an experiment similar to James Niederman's study at Yale. One group of entering students who had not been infected with EBV would be given the EBV vaccine. Then he would compare this group with a group of students who had not received the vaccine to see if there were fewer cases of mononucleosis in those vaccinated. If the vaccine is successful, it can be tried on children in Africa to prevent Burkitt's lymphoma and on adults in Southeast Asia and China where nasopharyngeal carcinoma is a problem. Testing the vaccine to prevent nasopharyngeal carcinoma would be much harder because this disease develops later in life, often many years after exposure to EBV.

Should Everyone Be Vaccinated Against EBV?

Scientists have no doubt that a vaccine against EBV would be a good thing for people living in Africa and other places where lymphoma and other serious EBV-associated diseases are common. But is it a good idea to give a vaccine to prevent mono to the general public in the United States and other developed countries? "Is the persistent stimulation of the immune system by EBV somehow beneficial to the majority of the population? The fact that nearly all people have antibodies and T-cell-mediated response against EBV may be of some benefit," Dr. Morgan points out. "Does this provide also a broad immunity against other herpesvirus infections?"[8] That is a question that will need to be resolved when researchers have finished developing and testing effective vaccines against EBV.

Future Treatment Possibilities

Treatments are being explored to prevent EBV from causing lymphomas in people who are given immunosuppressant drugs for cancer or when receiving organ transplants. Interferon, for example, is a natural body substance that is produced by cells that have been infected by a virus. It helps to protect other cells from infection. Researchers have developed methods for producing large amounts of interferon and have been testing its effects against various viral diseases and cancer. Some patients who received interferon combined with intravenous immunoglobulin active against herpesviruses seemed to benefit when it was given early in infection or prophylactically before they became infected with EBV. But it didn't help other patients, and it also interfered with the immunosuppressive therapy.[9]

Antiviral drugs such as acyclovir, ganciclovir, zidovudine (AZT), and foscarnet have been effective against EBV in cell cultures. But tests on human mono patients have not been as promising. Acyclovir, for example, did stop viral shedding, but the effect was only temporary and disappeared as soon as the patients stopped taking the drug. And there was no significant improvement in the patients' symptoms.

Treatment approaches using interleukin-2 are also being pursued. In laboratory experiments interleukin-2 prevented EBV-infected B cells from reproducing. It showed specific suppressor or killer activity against EBV-infected B cells.[10] But considering that some studies have implicated interleukin-2 in chronic fatigue syndrome, careful studies will be needed to determine whether this treatment approach is promising.

Various avenues of treatment for infectious mononucleosis and other EBV-associated illnesses are being pursued in many laboratories around the world. The insights and discoveries that these studies are yielding will bring benefits not only in the treatment of mono but in the control of other viral diseases as well.

Q & A

Q. Why is mono called the "kissing disease"?

A. Because the main way that infectious mononucleosis is transmitted is by very close contact, permitting a transfer of saliva from an infected person, which can occur during kissing.

Q. What kind of germ causes mono?

A. The Epstein-Barr virus, a member of the herpesvirus family. About 10 percent of monolike illnesses are caused by another herpesvirus, called cytomegalovirus.

Q. Is that the herpes you can catch by having sex?

A. No. Herpes type 2 (genital herpes) is caused by a different member of the same virus family, which can infect the reproductive organs. EBV infects cells in the throat lining and certain types of white blood cells.

Q. The boy I sit next to in class is in the hospital with mono now. Am I going to catch it?

A. Probably not (unless you've been kissing him). There is a small possibility that he has passed the virus that causes mono to you by coughing or spraying saliva when he talked to you, or by sharing a drinking glass or a pen after he had put the end in his mouth. But there is a good chance you are already protected by a childhood virus infection that you don't even remember; and only about half of the unprotected people who become infected as teens and young adults actually develop mono.

Q. My cousin just got mono, but she says she has never even been near anybody who had it. How did she catch it?

A. The Epstein-Barr virus remains in the body, and sometimes it becomes active again. So she might have caught it from someone who was not sick at the time.

Q. My brother just got mono at college, and my dad won't let my little sister and me visit him in the hospital. Is he overreacting?

A. Probably. If you don't kiss your brother on the mouth and wash your hands after touching him or things he has used, there is not much chance of your catching mono from him.

Q. My uncle is HIV-positive, and he wouldn't come to visit me when I had mono. Was he overreacting?

A. No. The AIDS virus (HIV) damages people's immune defenses and makes them more vulnerable to infections. An EBV infection can cause cancer or other very serious complications in immune-compromised people.

Q. Is there more mono around than there used to be?

A. Yes. Until about a century ago, nearly everyone became infected with EBV in childhood, when symptoms are usually very mild. Higher sanitation standards and less crowded living conditions now protect many people from infection until the teen or young adult years, when mono is more likely to occur.

Q. I have a sore throat, I'm running a fever, and I feel tired. Do I have mono?

A. Maybe. A number of diseases have those symptoms, but there are quick blood tests for mono that your doctor may even be able to do in the office while you are there.

Q. If there's no cure for mono, and I'm just supposed to rest, gargle with salt water, and take acetaminophen, did I waste my money going to the doctor to get diagnosed?

A. No. First of all, would you rather be worrying about whether you have leukemia or some other serious disease? A mono diagnosis can relieve your mind. And, secondly, your doctor has warned you about precautions to take and warning signs of complications to watch for.

Mono Timeline

1880s—German doctors describe "glandular fever."

1920—Thomas P. Sprunt and Frank A. Evans use the term "infectious mononucleosis" to describe the disease and distinguish it from leukemia.

1932—John R. Paul and Walls W. Bunnell devise the heterophile agglutination test for mono.

1957—Denis Burkitt observes Burkitt's lymphoma in Africa.

1964—M. Anthony Epstein and Yvonne Barr observe Epstein-Barr virus (EBV) in the electron microscope.

1967—Werner and Gertrude Henle identify EBV in the blood of a mono patient.

1984—M. T. Biggin, P. J. Farrell, and their associates report the complete DNA sequence of an EBV virus and locate the gene for the gp340 protein.

1984—David, the "bubble boy," dies of lymphoma caused by EBV received in a bone marrow transplant.

1985—Chronic fatigue syndrome first makes headlines as "yuppie flu."

1988—CDC issues a case definition for chronic fatigue syndrome, and EBV is not mentioned.

1989—Kevin Moore and Tim Mosmann find an EBV gene similar to that for interleukin-10.

For More Information

American Liver Foundation
1425 Pompton Avenue
Cedar Grove, NJ 07009
(800) 223-0179
(Toll-free hot line)

Children's Liver Foundation
14245 Venture Boulevard,
Suite 201
Sherman Oaks, CA 91423

The CFIDS Association
P.O. Box 220398
Charlotte, NC 28222-0398
(800) 442-3437

Department of Health &
Human Services
Public Health Service
Centers for Disease Control
Atlanta, GA 30333

CFS Advisory Council
12105 E. 54th Terrace
Kansas City, MO 64133

National Institute of Allergy
and Infectious Diseases
National Institutes of Health
Bethesda, MD 20892

Children's Hospital of
Philadelphia
34th St. & Civic Center Blvd.
Philadelphia, PA 19104

Minann, Inc.
P.O. Box 582
Glenview, IL 60025

Chapter Notes

Chapter 1

1. Patricia Thomas, "When a Kiss Can Make You Sick," *World Book Health and Medical Annual,* 1990, p. 128.

2. Jo Cassidy, "What's in a Name? Mononucleosis," *Current Health 2,* (September 1990), p. 15.

3. Thomas, p. 129.

4. Evelyn Zamula, "In Camps & On Campuses 'Mono' Is Still Part of the Scene," *FDA Consumer* (March 1986), p. 24.

Chapter 2

1. Robert T. Schooley, "Etiology," *Infectious Mononucleosis* (New York: Springer-Verlag, 1989), p. 1.

2. Michael Halberstam, "The 'Kissing Disease' That Isn't So Romantic," *Today's Health* (December 1974), p. 46.

3. Peter Radetsky, *The Invisible Invaders* (Boston: Little, Brown, 1991), p. 166.

4. Ann Giudici Fettner, *Science of Viruses* (New York: Morrow, 1990), p. 120.

5. Radetsky, p. 166.

6. Patricia Thomas, "When a Kiss Can Make You Sick," *The World Book Health and Medical Annual,* 1990, p.129.

Chapter 3

1. Evelyn Zamula, "In Camps & On Campuses 'Mono' Is Still Part of the Scene," *FDA Consumer* (March 1986), p. 24.

2. Robert Berkow, ed., "Infectious Mononucleosis," *The Merck Manual* (Rahway, N.J.: Merck Sharp & Dohme, 1992), p. 2282.

3. Peter Radetsky, *The Invisible Invaders* (Boston: Little, Brown, 1991), p. 177.

4. Peter Axelrod and Albert Finestone, "Infectious Mononucleosis in Older Adults," *American Family Physician* (December 1990), p. 1601.

5. Ibid, p. 1600.

6. Stephen Straus and Gary Fleisher, "Infectious Mononucleosis Epidemiology and Pathogenesis," in *Infectious Mononucleosis* (New York: Springer-Verlag, 1989), p. 14.

7. Ibid.

8. Ibid., p. 16.

9. Zamula, p. 24.

10. Abram S. Benenson, ed., *Control of Communicable Diseases in Man* (Washington, D.C.: American Public Health Association, 1990), p. 292.

11. Berkow, p. 2281.

12. Patricia Thomas, "When a Kiss Can Make You Sick," *The World Book Health and Medical Annual,* 1990, p. 133.

13. Berkow, p. 2281.

14. Radetsky, p. 177.

15. Paul Chervenick, "Infectious Mononucleosis: The Classic Clinical Syndrome," *Infectious Mononucleosis* (New York: Springer-Verlag, 1989), p.14.

16. Benenson, p. 116.

17. Axelrod and Finestone, p. 1601.

18. Ibid.

Chapter 4

1. Patricia Thomas, "When a Kiss Can Make You Sick," *The World Book Health and Medical Annual,* 1990, p. 128.

2. "Backgrounder: Infectious Mononucleosis," pamphlet from the National Institute of Allergy and Infectious Disease (April 1992), p. 3.

3. Peter Axelrod and Albert Finestone, "Infectious Mononucleosis in Older Adults," *American Family Physician* (December 1990), p. 1600.

4. Ibid., pp. 1604–1605.

5. "Health Care the Oregon Way," *New York Times,* March 20, 1993, p. 20.

Chapter 5

1. Michael Halberstam, "The 'Kissing Disease' That Isn't So Romantic," *Today's Health* (December 1974), p. 46.

2. Zamula, "In Camps & On Campuses 'Mono' Is Still Part of the Scene," *FDA Consumer* (March 1986), p. 24.

3. J. Martin Kaplan, Marc Keller, and Shoshona Troy, "Nasopharyngeal Obstruction in Infectious Mononucleosis," *American Family Physician* (January 1987), p. 209.

4. "Backgrounder: Infectious Mononucleosis," pamphlet from the National Institute of Allergy and Infectious Disease (April 1992), p. 3.

5. Stephen E. Straus, moderator, "Epstein-Barr Virus Infections: Biology, Pathogenesis, and Management," *Annals of Internal Medicine* (January 1993), p. 55.

6. Ibid.

Chapter 6

1. J. Martin Kaplan, Marc Keller, and Shoshona Troy, "Nasopharyngeal Obstruction in Infectious Mononucleosis," *American Family Physician* (January 1987), p. 205.

2. Evelyn Zamula, "In Camps & On Campuses 'Mono' Is Still Part of the Scene," *FDA Consumer* (March 1986), p. 24.

3. Kaplan, Keller, and Troy, p. 205.

4. Ibid., p 209.

5. Peter Radetsky, *The Invisible Invaders* (Boston: Little, Brown, 1991), p. 177.

6. Morag C. Timbury, *Medical Virology* (New York: Churchill Livingstone, 1991), p. 109.

7. Joseph Pagano, "Epstein-Barr Virus: Culprit or Consort?" *The New England Journal of Medicine* (December 10, 1992), p. 1751.

8. T. Aya, "Chromosome Translocation and c-MYC Activation by Epstein-Barr Virus and Euphorbia Tirucalli in B Lymphocytes," *The Lancet* (May 18, 1991), p. 1190.

9. Andrew J. Morgan, "Control of Viral Disease: The Development of Epstein-Barr Virus Vaccines," *Springer Seminars in Immunopathology* (1991), pp. 249–262.

10. Sean Henahan, "Ready EBV Anticancer Vaccine for Clinical Trials in UK Volunteers," *Medical Tribune* (March 9, 1989), p. 12.

11. G. Pallesen, "Expression of Epstein-Barr Virus Latent Gene Products in Tumor Cells of Hodgkin's Disease," *The Lancet* (February 9, 1991), pp. 320–322.

12. R. S. Chang, *Infectious Mononucleosis* (Boston: G. K. Hall Medical Publishers, 1980), p. 144.

13. Clare Sample, "Molecular Basis For Epstein-Barr Virus Induced Pathogenesis and Disease," *Springer Seminars in Immunopathology* (1991), pp. 133–146.

14. Ian Magrath, "Infectious Mononucleosis and Malignant Neoplasia," in *Infectious Mononucleosis* (New York: Springer-Verlag, 1989), p. 162.

15. Chang, p. 148.

16. Robert Fox, "Reactivation of Epstein-Barr Virus in Sjögren's Syndrome," *Springer Seminars In Immunopathology* (1991), p. 217.

17. Radetsky, pp. 182–183.

18. Kenneth Culver, "Splice of Life," *The Sciences* (January/February 1993), p. 20.

19. Tadamasa Ooka, "Relationship Between Antibody Production to Epstein-Barr Virus (EBV) Early Antigens and Various EBV-Related Diseases," *Springer Seminars in Immunopathology* (1991), pp. 233–247.

20. Pagano, pp. 1750–1751.

Chapter 7

1. Peter Radetsky, *The Invisible Invaders* (Boston: Little, Brown, 1991), p. 156.

2. Pat Phillips, "Viral 'Team' Suspected in CFS," *Medical World News* (November 1991), p. 19.

3. Joseph Palca, "Does a Retrovirus Explain Fatigue Syndrome Puzzle?" *Science* (September 14, 1990), p. 1240.

4. Geoffrey Cowley, "Chronic Fatigue Syndrome," *Newsweek* (November 12, 1990), p. 64.

5. Max Gates, "Progress Reported On Fatigue Syndrome," *Star-Ledger* (Newark, N.J.), August 8, 1991, p. 49.

6. "Chronic Fatigue Syndrome," *American Family Physician* (February 1992), p. 933.

7. Phillips, p. 18.

8. Palca, "Does A Retrovirus Explain Fatigue Syndrome Puzzle?" p. 1241.

9. Joseph Palca, "On the Track of an Elusive Disease," *Science* (December 20, 1991), p. 1726.

10. Ron Winslow, "Chronic Fatigue Study Points To Herpes Virus," *The Wall Street Journal*, January 15, 1992, p. B5.

11. Palca, "On the Track of an Elusive Disease," pp. 1726–1727.

12. Jane E. Brody, "Chronic Fatigue Syndrome: How To Recognize It and What To Do About It," *New York Times*, July 28, 1988, p. B6.

13. Cowley, p. 69.

14. Jean Carper, "Immunology Research Links Food Allergies To Chronic Fatigue Syndrome," *Star-Ledger* (Newark, N.J.), September 9, 1992, p. 47.

15. Palca, "On the Track of an Elusive Disease," p. 1726.

16. Cowley, p. 62.

17. Palca, "On the Track of an Elusive Disease," p. 1726.

18. Cowley, p. 62.

Chapter 8

1. Marcia Barinaga, "Viruses Launch Their Own 'Star Wars'," *Science* (December 11, 1992), p. 1731.

2. Lindsey Hutt-Fletcher, "Epstein-Barr Virus Tissue Tropism" *Springer Seminars in Immunopathology* (1991), pp. 117–131.

3. Peter Radetsky, *The Invisible Invaders* (Boston: Little, Brown, 1991), p. 18.

4. Sean Henahan, "Ready EBV Anticancer Vaccine for Clinical Trials in UK Volunteers," *Medical Tribune* (March 9, 1989), p. 12.

5. Andrew J. Morgan, "Epstein-Barr Virus Vaccines," *Vaccine* Vol. 10, Issue 9, 1992, p. 563.

6. Andrew J. Morgan, "Control of Viral Disease: The Development of Epstein-Barr Virus Vaccines," *Springer Seminars in Immunopathology* (1991), pp. 249–262.

7. Ibid., p. 255.

8. Ibid., p. 258.

9. Ian Magrath, "Infectious Mononucleosis and Malignant Neoplasia," *Infectious Mononucleosis* (New York: Springer-Verlag, 1989), p. 157.

10. Ibid.

Glossary

AIDS—An acronym for Acquired Immune Deficiency Syndrome, a serious viral disease.

antibodies—Proteins produced to bind specifically to foreign chemicals (antigens), such as surface chemicals on an invading virus.

Burkitt's lymphoma—A cancer of the lymphatic system, linked with EBV.

carrier—A person infected with a disease microbe who, without showing any symptoms, can transmit the disease to others.

chronic fatigue syndrome—A long-lasting illness (or group of illnesses) whose cause is currently unknown but may be linked with EBV and/or other viruses. Also called chronic fatigue immune dysfunction syndrome.

corticosteroids—Adrenal hormones with anti-inflammatory effects.

cytomegalovirus—A common virus of the herpes family that can cause mononucleosis and liver damage.

encephalitis—Inflammation of the brain.

epithelial cells—Cells that form coverings and linings of body structures such as the skin and the mucous membranes lining the breathing passages.

Epstein-Barr virus (EBV)—A virus of the herpes family that causes mononucleosis and may damage the liver.

glycoprotein—A protein that contains sugars.

Guillain-Barré syndrome—A rare complication of mononucleosis involving weakness and sometimes paralysis of the leg and arm muscles.

hairy leukoplakia—An EBV infection of the surface of the tongue.

hemolytic anemia—A massive destruction of red blood cells.

hepatitis—Inflammation of the liver.

herpesvirus—One of a family of viruses including those that cause chicken pox, cold sores, mononucleosis, and genital herpes.

heterophile agglutination test—A reaction of antibodies to Epstein-Barr virus with antigens from sheep or horse blood, causing the red blood cells to "clump" (gather together into irregular masses).

heterophile antibodies—Antibodies produced against cells of a different species.

Hodgkin's disease—A lymphoma (cancer of the lymphatic system) linked with EBV infection.

immune system—A system of various body defenses against invading microbes, including white blood cells and interferon.

immunity—The ability to resist a disease through the action of disease-fighting cells adapted to attack an invading microbe or its products.

incubation period—The time between infection with a virus or bacterium and the appearance of symptoms of disease.

inflammation—Swelling, pain, heat, and redness in the tissues around a site of infection.

interferon—A protein released by virus-infected cells that protects other cells from infection.

interleukins—Substances that regulate immune system functions.

jaundice—A yellowing of the skin and the whites of the eyes due to a buildup of bile pigments in the blood and tissues.

"kissing disease"—A popular name for infectious mononucleosis, reflecting one of its major transmission routes.

latent infection—An infection in which the germ is currently inactive and no symptoms are evident.

leukemia—Cancer of the blood-forming tissues; one of the early symptoms is an abnormally large number of mononuclear lymphocytes.

lymph nodes—Organs of the immune system, in which disease-fighting white blood cells congregate. Popularly called "glands," they are found in various parts of the body, including the neck, armpits, and groin.

lymphocytes—Disease-fighting white blood cells. Some produce antibodies; other types attack foreign or cancer cells or produce immune-regulating chemicals.

meningitis—An inflammation of the meninges, the membranes covering the brain and spinal cord.

mono—The popular name for infectious mononucleosis, a highly contagious viral disease caused mainly by the Epstein-Barr virus.

mononuclear lymphocytes—Disease-fighting white blood cells with a single nucleus that can become macrophages, large amoeba-like cells that engulf and digest microbes. Also called **monocytes**.

Monospot test—A heterophile antibody test used to diagnose infectious mononucleosis.

nasopharyngeal carcinoma—Cancer of the nose and throat.

Paul-Bunnell antibodies—Heterophile antibodies, the presence of which indicates active EBV infection.

Purtilo's syndrome—A hereditary disorder in which a person has no defenses against EBV infection. Also called X-linked lymphoproliferative syndrome.

severe combined immunodeficiency (SCID)—A hereditary disorder in which disease-fighting lymphocytes are not produced. Sometimes called "bubble-boy disease," after a widely publicized case.

Sjögren's syndrome—An autoimmune disease characterized by severe dryness of the eyes and mouth.

spleen—A large abdominal organ that acts as a reservoir for blood and also contains cells and tissues of the immune system.

swollen glands—Inflamed lymph nodes. (Not really "glands," which are organs that secrete hormones, digestive enzymes, or other products.)

throat culture—A test for strep throat (an infection caused by Streptococcus bacteria) in which secretions are taken from the throat with a cotton swab. The secretions are then applied to a culture dish on which bacteria multiply to form visible colonies.

thrombocytopenia—A lack of blood platelets (blood components that help in blood clotting).

tonsils—Masses of lymph tissue in the throat, which become enlarged and inflamed when white blood cells are actively fighting an infection.

tracheostomy—A temporary opening in the throat made surgically to permit air to bypass an obstruction of the upper breathing passages.

vaccination—Administration (usually by injection or orally) of a preparation of microbes or their products to stimulate protective immunity against disease.

vaccinia—An attenuated (weakened) virus formerly used for smallpox vaccinations and now being used as a part of genetically engineered vaccines.

Further Reading

Books

Fettner, Ann Guidici. *Science of Viruses.* New York: Morrow, 1990.

Radetsky, Peter. *The Invisible Invaders.* Boston: Little, Brown, 1991.

Schlossberg, David, ed. *Infectious Mononucleosis* (2nd ed.). New York: Springer-Verlag, 1989.

Articles

Axelrod, Peter and Albert J. Finestone. "Infectious Mononucleosis in Older Adults." *American Family Physician,* December 1990, pp. 1599–1606.

Barinaga, Marcia. "Viruses Launch Their Own 'Star Wars'. *Science,* December 11, 1992, pp. 1731–1732.

Brody, Jane E. "Chronic Fatigue Syndrome: How To Recognize It and What To Do About It." *New York Times,* July 28, 1988, p. B6.

Cassidy, Jo. "What's In a Name? Mononucleosis." *Current Health 2,* September 1990, pp. 14–15.

Cherfas, Jeremy. "Chronic Fatigue as Chameleon." *Science,* September 14, 1990, p. 1240.

Cowley, Geoffrey, Mary Hager, and Nadine Joseph. "Chronic Fatigue Syndrome." *Newsweek,* November 12, 1990, pp. 62–70.

Dinsmoor, Robert. "When Mono Attacks, Take It Lying Down." *Current Health 2,* September 1993, pp. 30–31.

Halberstam, Michael. "The 'Kissing Disease' That Isn't So Romantic." *Today's Health,* December 1974, pp. 44–47.

Jennings, Karla. "Hodgkin's Disease: The Cancer That Hits Young Women Hardest." *Cosmopolitan,* October 1991, pp. 172, 176.

Kaplan, J. Martin, Marc S. Keller, and Shoshona Troy. "Nasopharyngeal Obstruction in Infectious Mononucleosis." *American Family Physician,* January 1987, pp. 205–209.

"More Than Just a Kissing Disease." *Glamour,* March 1980, pp. 256, 258.

Morgan, Andrew J. "Epstein-Barr Virus Vaccines." *Vaccine,* Vol. 10, Issue 9, 1992, pp. 563–571.

Okano, Motohiko, Geoffrey M. Thiele, and David T. Purtilo. "Update on Mononucleosis and Other EBV Infections." *Diagnosis,* January 1989, pp. 12–18.

Pagano, Joseph S. "Epstein-Barr Virus: Culprit or Consort?" *The New England Journal of Medicine,* December 10, 1992, pp. 1750–1752.

Palca, Joseph. "Does a Retrovirus Explain Fatigue Syndrome Puzzle?" *Science,* September 14, 1990, pp. 1240–1241.

Palca, Joseph. "On the Track of an Elusive Disease." *Science,* December 20, 1991, pp. 1726–1728.

Straus, Stephen E., moderator, "Epstein-Barr Virus Infections: Biology, Pathogenesis, and Management." *Annals of Internal Medicine,* January 1993, pp. 45–58.

Suyama, Ciro V. "Mononucleosis in Children: An Update." *Patient Care,* November 15, 1990, pp. 139–158.

Thomas, Patricia. "Mono: When a Kiss Can Make You Sick." *The World Book Health & Medical Annual 1990,* pp. 127–139.

Zamula, Evelyn. "In Camps & On Campus 'Mono' Is Still Part of the Scene." *FDA Consumer,* March 1986, pp. 23–25.

Index

111